Images of Modern America

KINGS PARK PSYCHIATRIC CENTER

On the Front Cover: This photograph was taken in Building 93. (Courtesy of Tammy Rebello and TMR Visual Arts.)

On the Back Cover: The photograph of the benches was taken outside the surgical center, and the other three were taken inside Building 93. (Courtesy of Tammy Rebello and TMR Visual Arts.)

Images of Modern America

KINGS PARK PSYCHIATRIC CENTER

L.F. Blanchard and Tammy Rebello
Foreword by Leo P. Ostebo and JoAnn Galletta Hahn

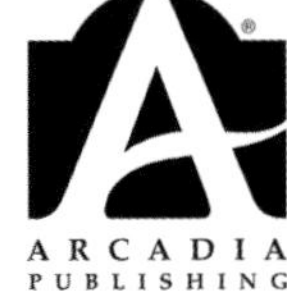

ISBN 978-1-4671-0287-2

Published by Arcadia Publishing
Charleston, South Carolina

Printed in the United States of America

Library of Congress Control Number: 2018968224

For all general information, please contact Arcadia Publishing:
Telephone 843-853-2070
Fax 843-853-0044
E-mail sales@arcadiapublishing.com
For customer service and orders:
Toll-Free 1-888-313-2665

Visit us on the Internet at www.arcadiapublishing.com

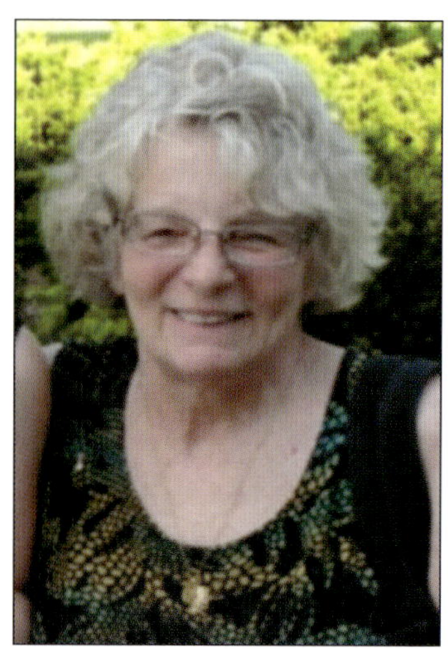

Lynn and Tammy dedicate this book in loving memory of our friend and No. 1 fan and cheerleader, Peggy Zuckerman. Thank you for always believing in us, and the love and light you shared at every encounter. You are truly missed.

Tammy dedicates this book in loving memory of Shiloh "Shi" Murphy. Shiloh died by suicide after a battle with depression at the young age of 16. She will forever be a bright light in our lives. Shi is loved and missed beyond words. Be free, beautiful girl.

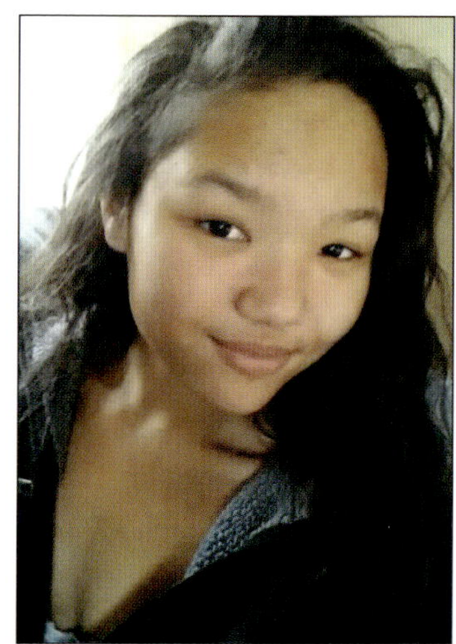

CONTENTS

Foreword

Kings Park State Hospital was deeply influential in the growth of the town of Kings Park for over 110 years. Before the town was truly established, its beginnings were established around St. Johnland, established by the Episcopal minister Dr. Rev. William Augustus Muhlenberg in 1866. After Muhlenberg established St. Luke's Hospital in New York City, his vision was to form a serene park setting on the north shore of Long Island, an attempt to move families, crippled orphans, and the elderly far from the urban squalor of the city. In 1872, the railroad came into the area bringing visitors and necessary goods, and the local stop was known as St. Johnland. Years after Kings Park State Hospital was established and growing, the railroad officially named the station Kings Park in June 1891 and the town was officially rooted.

In 1994, the state initiated plans to close the hospital. With a gathering of some high school students, retired KPHS English/history teacher Leo Ostebo, and two other townspeople, the idea of having a heritage museum began, based on the closing of one of the country's largest, oldest, and most medically significant occupational therapy mental hospitals.

The Kings Park Heritage Museum is the only school community–managed museum in the United States and is the result of over 25 years of continuous efforts.

—Leo P. Ostebo, Museum Curator and Director
Joann Galletta Hahn, Board of Trustees President

Acknowledgments

Our thanks go to Tina Runyan, PhD, for her constant support, unwavering faith, and inspiration of #BeTheLight.

A huge thank-you is extended to the fine folks at the Leo P. Ostebo Kings Park Heritage Museum—Leo P. Ostebo and Joann Galletta Hahn, for her constant support and always being available to answer our questions and offer her amazing support; David Flynn, for sharing his extensive knowledge; Dr. George Tiernan; and the residents of Kings Park for their hospitality and for sharing their stories.

We would also like to acknowledge all the libraries, bookstores (big and small), the local shops who helped us spread the word, and galleries who welcomed us to tell our story, all the radio, television, and newspaper reporters who helped spread the word, and all those who found the strength to share their own stories along the way.

Unless otherwise noted, all images are from Tammy Rebello and TMR Visual Arts.

Introduction

Among the most often asked questions we get is how we got started with this project and what drives us. Tammy and I have known each other for three decades, and while there was a time when we had lost touch, busy in our own lives, we reconnected on Facebook several years ago. Tammy had been photographing for over 20 years at that time, and on a whim, based on the interest her kids took in an episode of *Ghost Adventures*, she grabbed her camera and headed out to the New York location. While exploring, she discovered a strong desire to tell the story of these places. This is when she came to me.

We approached this project from different angles. Tammy loved the architecture, the style of the buildings, and the artistry of the physical structure set against the rubble left behind. She recently told me how much it saddens her to see these places being torn down. If perhaps they had taken care of these buildings instead of letting them rot, they could have been saved for future generations to see how beautiful they truly are.

Being a therapist, I came at it from the psychological perspective. I wanted to know for what purpose the facilities were built, what they became, and what led to their demise. I explored the story with the perspective of the state, the institution and administrators, employees, patients, and their loved ones. I am interested in story of how the mental health field in Massachusetts, Connecticut, New York, and the United States changed over the past century, and why.

Our goal has always been to tell the story, to let you in behind the scenes; to perhaps, in our own way, start to change the stigma associated with mental illness. While we have come so far in this field, we still have a battle ahead. For those working to better the lives of others, who teach the tools to a more peaceful state of mind, I commend you. But to those who struggle, you are not alone. Both Tammy and I found the courage to step into the light, and you can too. #BeTheLight

One

In the Beginning

Kings Park has always been different. From the 1890s and through much of the 20th century, Kings Park was largely Democratic, Irish, Roman Catholic, and Jewish when most of Long Island was Republican, English, and Protestant. Kings Park, established in 1891, was a company town. That company, however, did not make cars or mine coal; it was the Kings Park State Hospital (1885–1996), which was established as a replacement for the overcrowded Kings County Asylum in Brooklyn. As the hospital grew, the town grew, and generations of culturally diverse families and residents worked at the state hospital until it closed. The town developed and flourished through the years, becoming and continuing to be the tight-knit community it is today. It is difficult to imagine a built-up place more beautiful and idyllic than the hospital. Its location along the north shore of Long Island Sound and the Nissequogue River made the hospital a perfect, peaceful setting. It was a visually impressive campus inside and out that few people were fortunate enough to see and experience, paired with a historic town that grew strong alongside.

—David Flynn
Kings Park Resident,
Town of Smithtown Planning Director (1980–2018)
Museum Assistant Director
(David's parents were both nurses at the Kings Park State Hospital.)

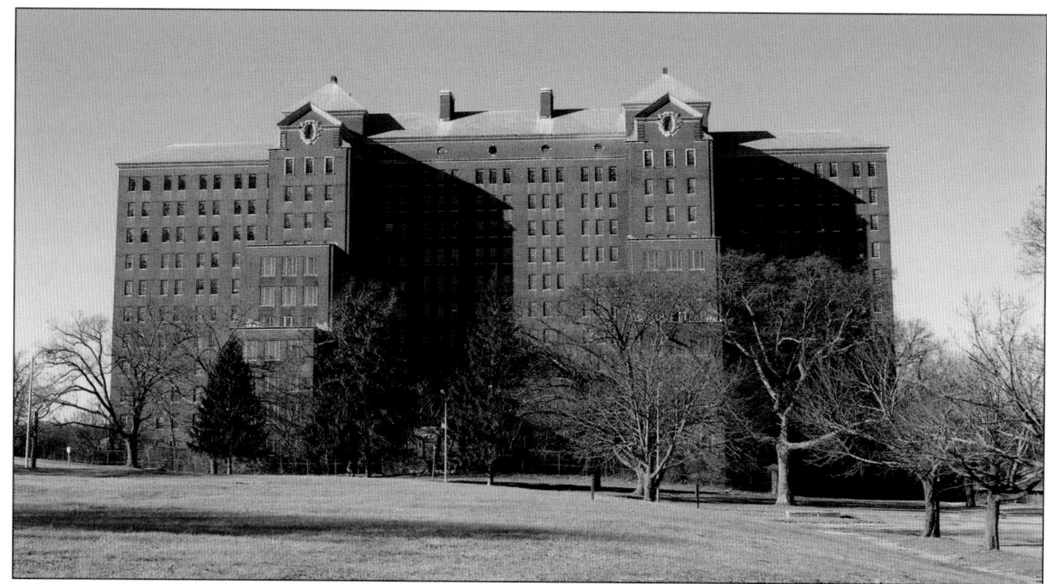

While not the first to open state-supported facilities specifically for those suffering from mental illness, New York State has been an innovator in development, treatment, and research in the field. New York was, however the first to make the care of these individuals solely the responsibility of the state, rather than the cities and counties, via the 1890 State Care Act. The following photographs were taken on Wards 17–38.

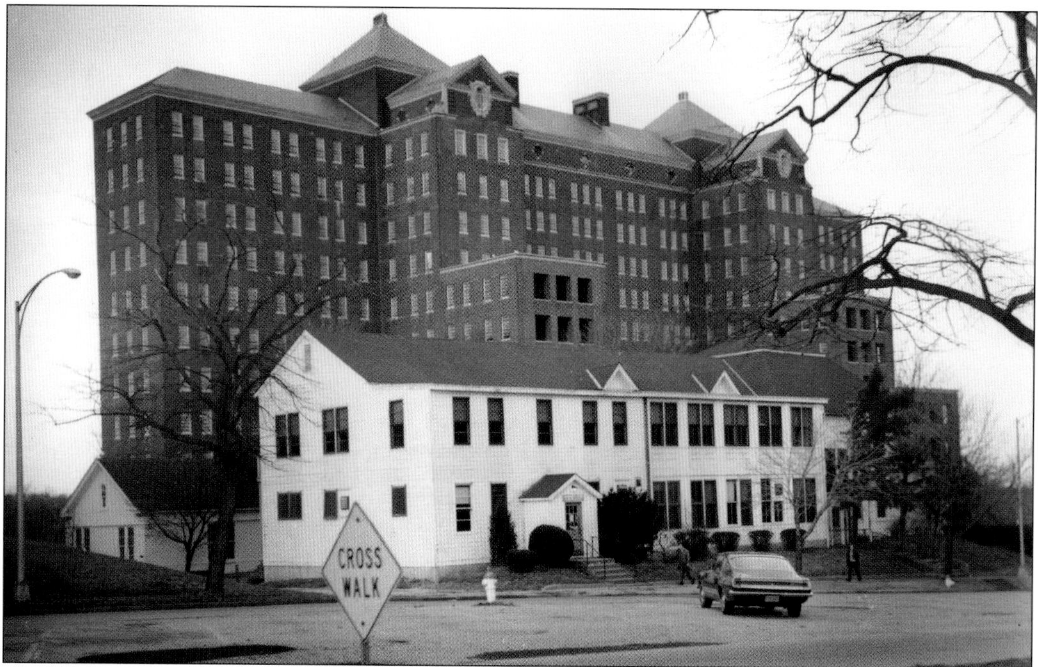

Shown here is the Continuing Treatment building. Opening its doors in 1885, Kings County Asylum, later renamed Kings Park Psychiatric Hospital, was built to alleviate overcrowded hospitals within the Kings County limits. Like many of its time, it was considered a farm colony, meaning it put patients to work tending livestock and growing their own food as a form of therapy. (Courtesy of the Leo P. Ostebo Kings Park Heritage Museum.)

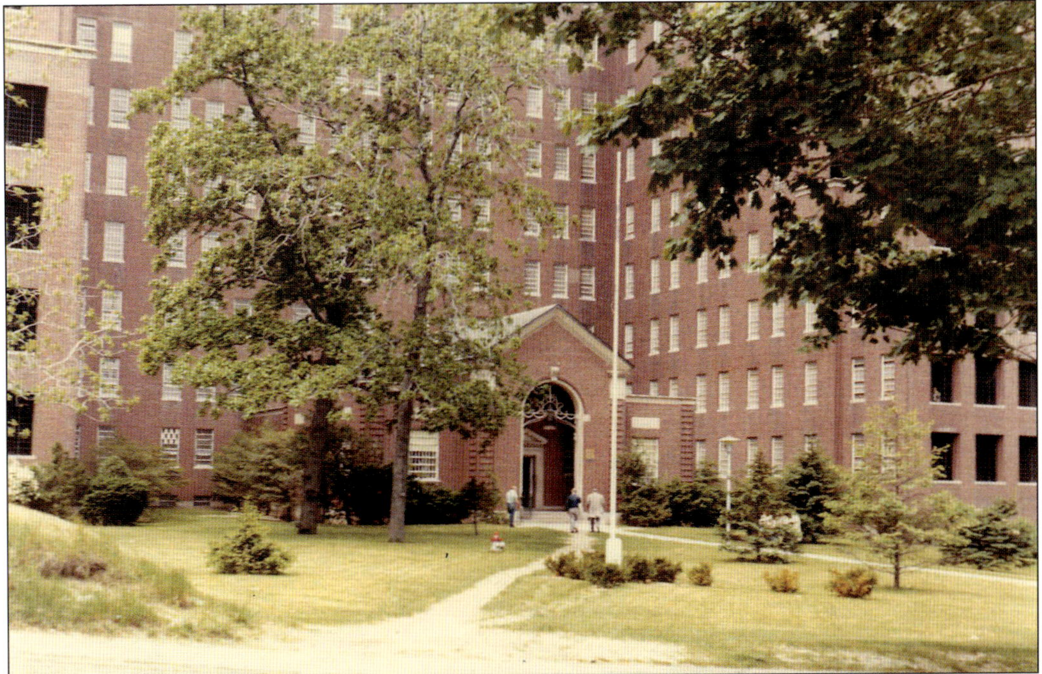

It was also built in a more colony-style layout, with the intention of it feeling more "homelike" to the residents and staff. The farm work helped keep costs down, as well as giving the patients a sense of purpose, keeping them occupied and satiated. (Courtesy of the Leo P. Ostebo Kings Park Heritage Museum.)

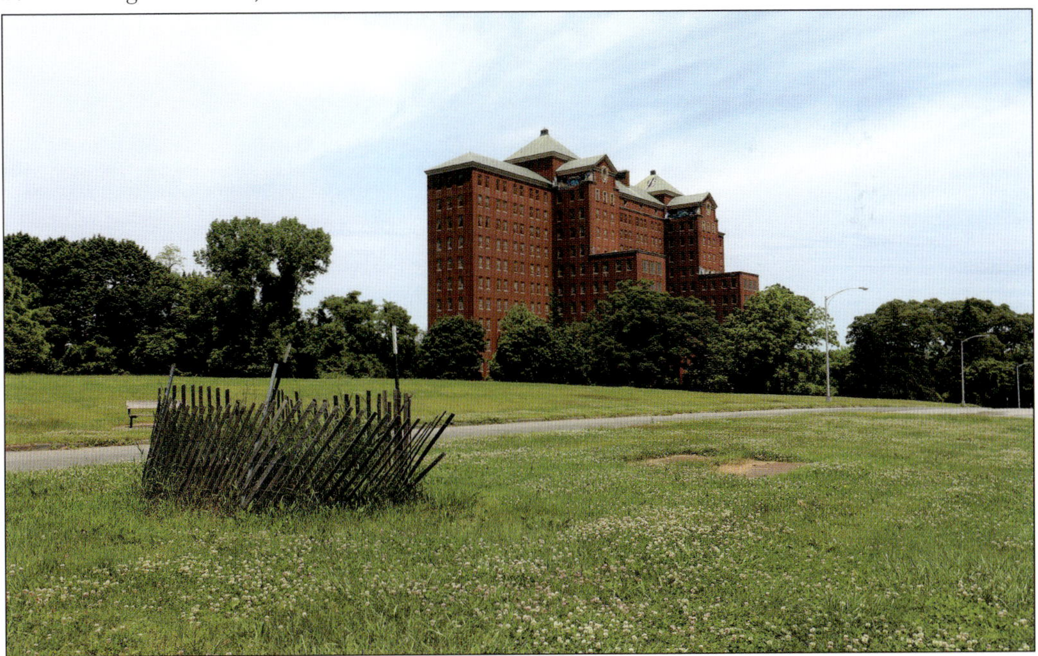

Kings Park Psychiatric Center tried to avoid the high-rise model of many of the asylums of the day, with the general feeling that it was not as humane or comfortable for the patients. However, in 1939, it did become necessary to build a 13-story structure, Building 93.

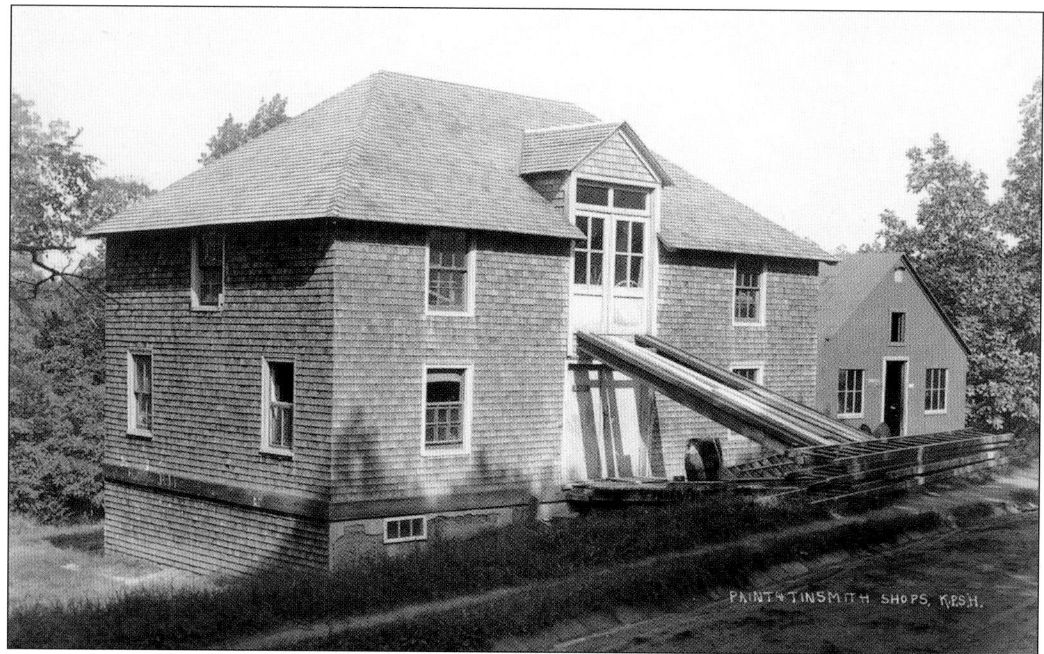

This was intended to help keep up with the high demand for placements for patients and the boom of the New York City area in the 1930s. By the 1950s, the facility had over 100 buildings, including power plants, fire stations, staff housing, hospitals, recreational facilities, piggeries, and cow barns. (Courtesy of the Leo P. Ostebo Kings Park Heritage Museum.)

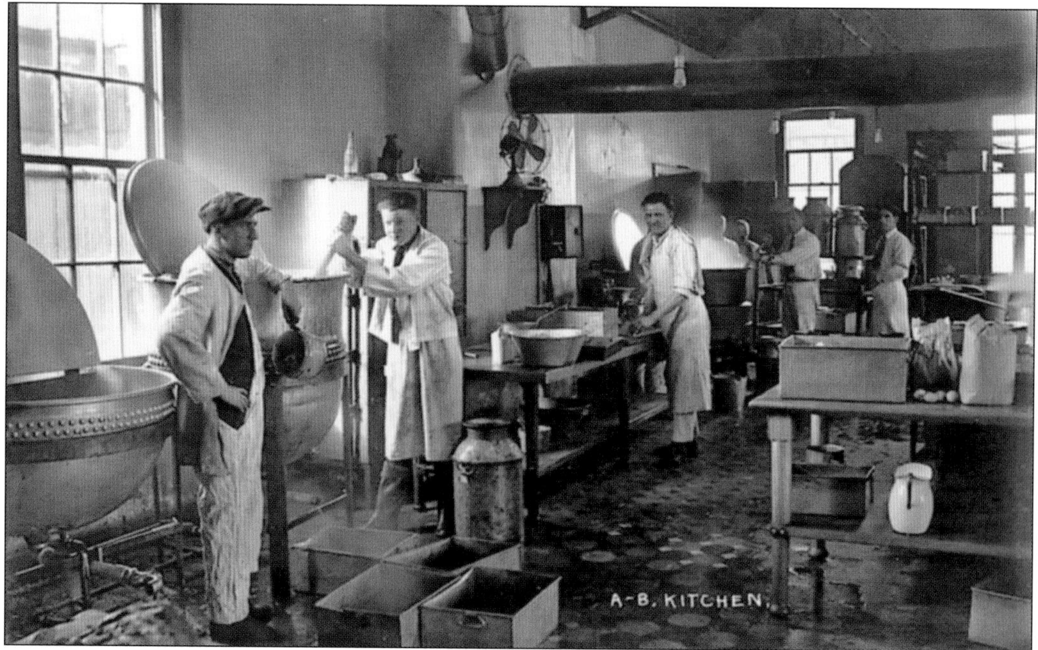

The population peaked at the hospital in 1954 with 9,303 patients, which meant an increasing need for staff. This in turn drove the development of the town. Kings Park, situated on the north shore of Long Island, offered many of the staff and their families a new community closer to work. (Courtesy of the Leo P. Ostebo Kings Park Heritage Museum.)

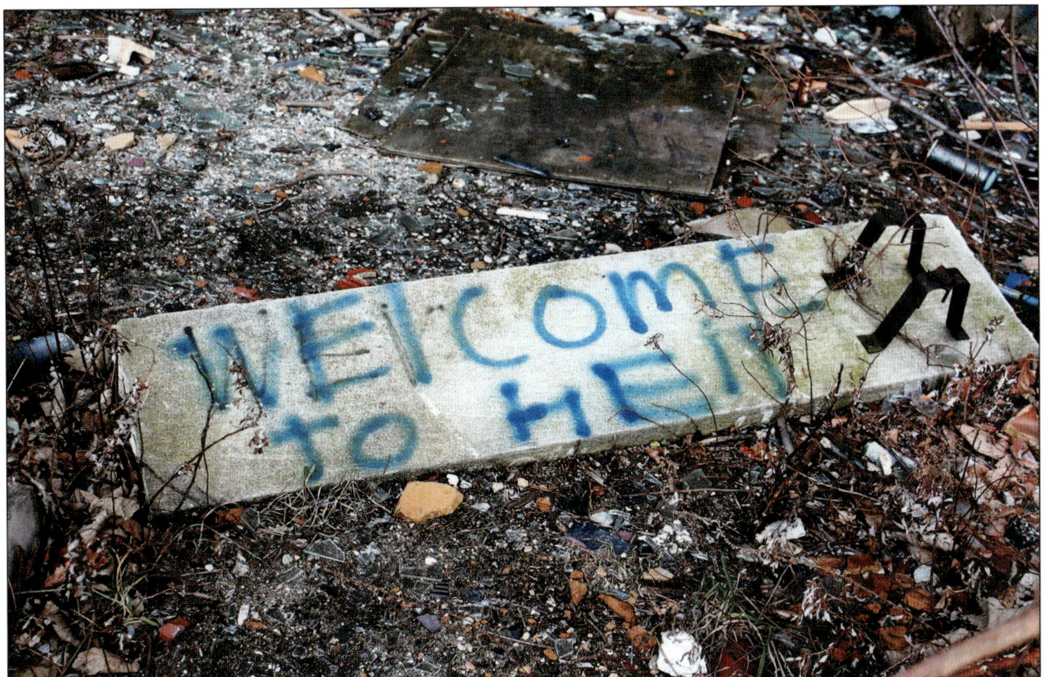

Throughout the facility of over 100 buildings, the residents were organized by gender, age, temperament, and physical limitation. In 1996, Kings Park's last residents were relocated to nearby Pilgrim State Hospital. Kings Park Psychiatric Hospital was well known for being innovative in the field of psychological science.

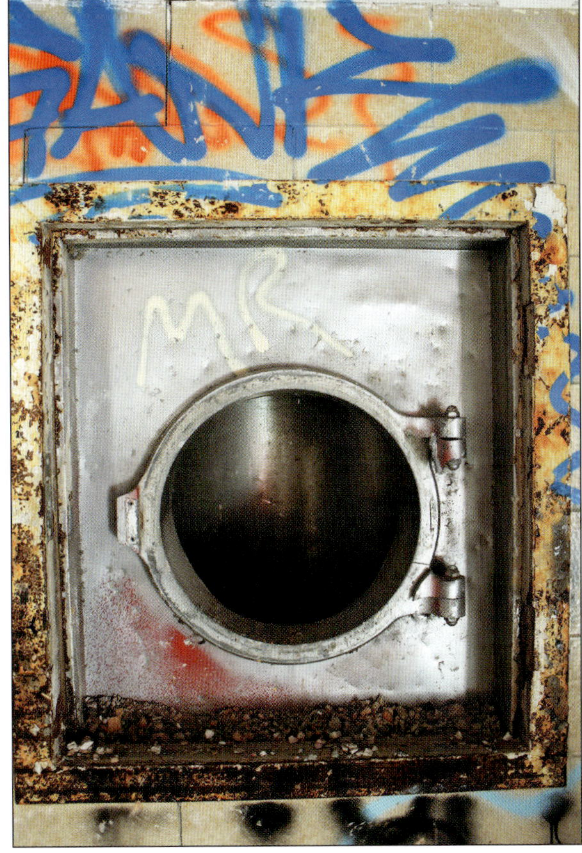

While often working with the newest procedures and medications, such as the prefrontal lobotomy, this modernization may have led to its downfall. While at the time thought to be innovative, the lobotomy is considered by many to be barbaric. The procedure, which has also been referred to as a leucotomy, or leukotomy, is a neurological operation intended to sever the connections in the brain's prefrontal lobe.

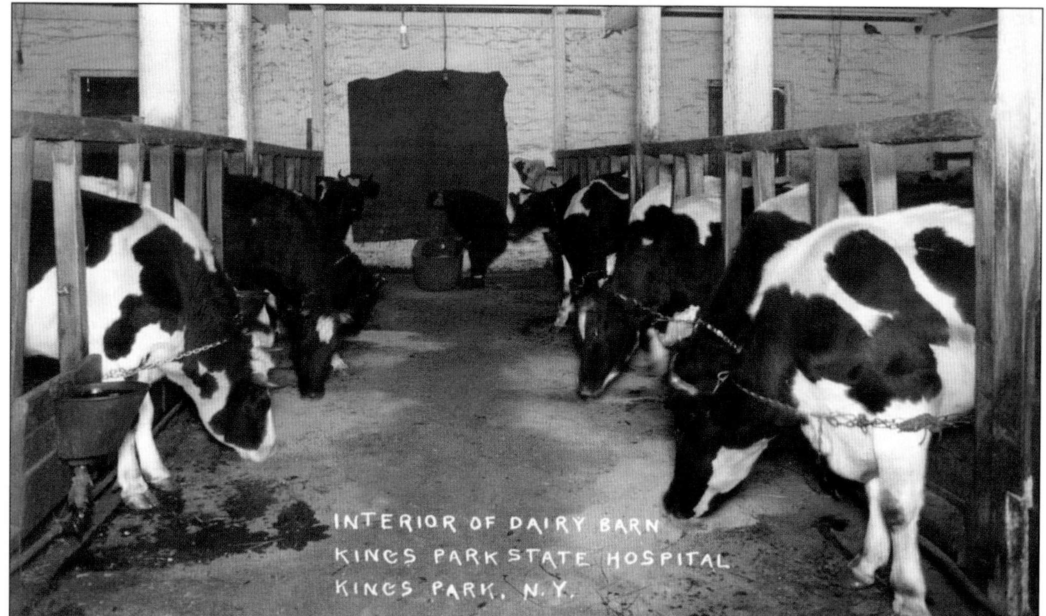

A mental probe was inserted through the eye socket into the brain cavity and moved back and forth to sever the connections of the prefrontal cortex from the rest of the brain. The thinking of the time was that if doctors could fix the neurological connections between the frontal lobe and the rest of the brain, they could stop undesirable behaviors. (Courtesy of the Leo P. Ostebo Kings Park Heritage Museum.)

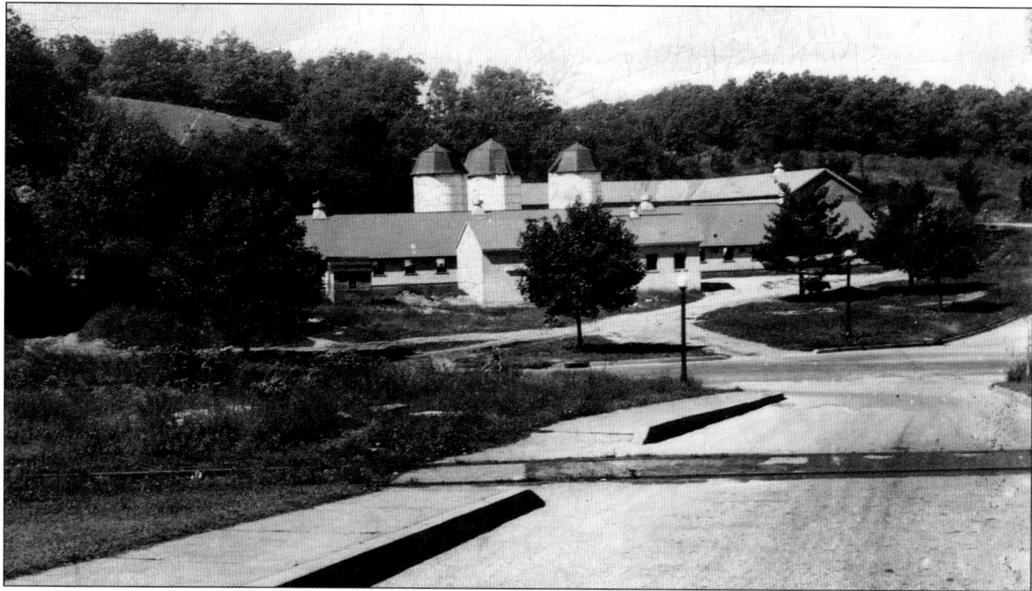

Lobotomies were commonly used for the treatment of schizophrenia, manic depression, panic disorder, mania, and bipolar disorder. Unfortunately, these operations came at a high cost, with adverse side effects such as incontinence, vomiting, eating disorders, lethargy, apathy, epilepsy, loss of motor function, loss of cognitive abilities, paralysis, and death. This photograph shows the farm building on the campus of the facility. (Courtesy of the Leo P. Ostebo Kings Park Heritage Museum.)

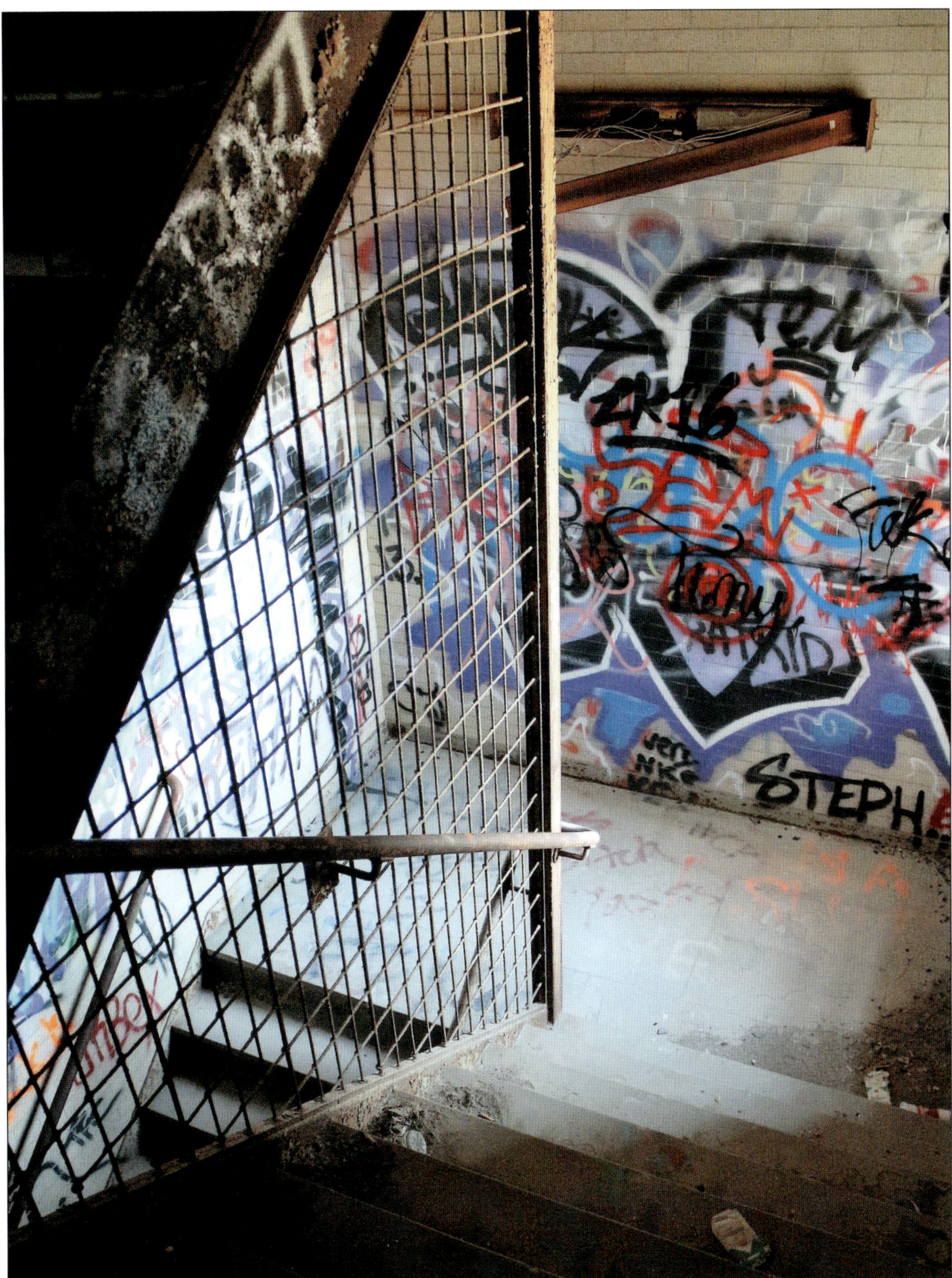

Prior to the release of antipsychotic and antidepressant medications, lobotomies were used to treat different types of mental illness. Lobotomies became a common treatment for conditions like severe depression, schizophrenia, and suicidal ideations. These were considered viable options for treatment. In the 1950s, with the advent of antipsychotics, the field of mental health care began to change, many felt for the better.

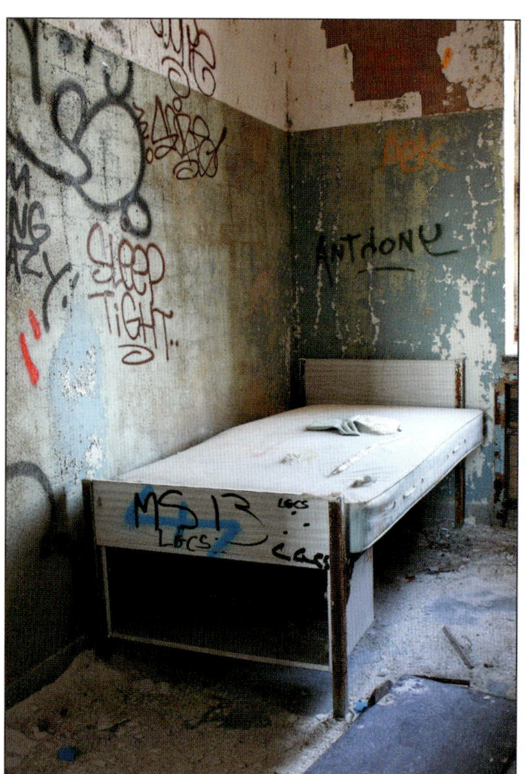

Though it would take many years before the full benefits were seen, these new medications offered hope to patients as an alternative to the brutality of lobotomies, shock treatments, ice baths, and seclusion.

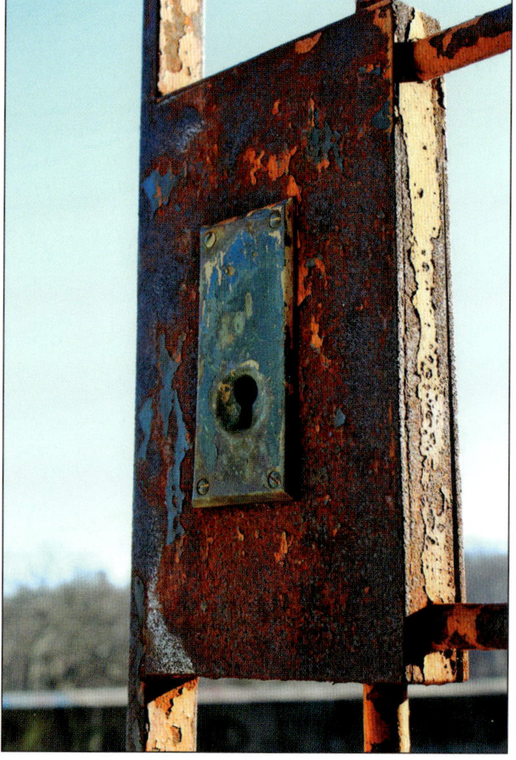

These medications, and those that followed, made it possible for patients to be effectively treated with outpatient services, which increased in the coming decades. In 1996, Kings Park Psychiatric Hospital ended its 111-year run. A facility that was once severely overcrowded and understaffed quickly emptied, as it had become nearly obsolete.

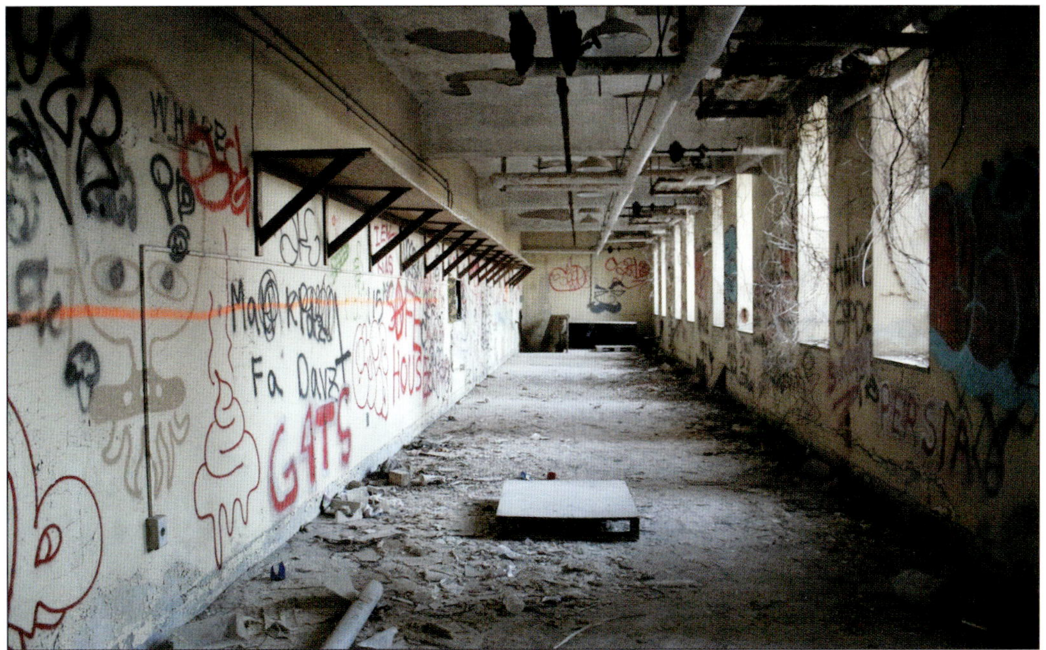

Sam, a Kings Park Psychiatric Center employee, recalled that when he first went to work at "the Psych Center," as the locals came to call it, he was barely 18. He had neatly pressed his white suit and arrived early for his first shift, despite his fears. He described the experience of his first time on the floor as scary.

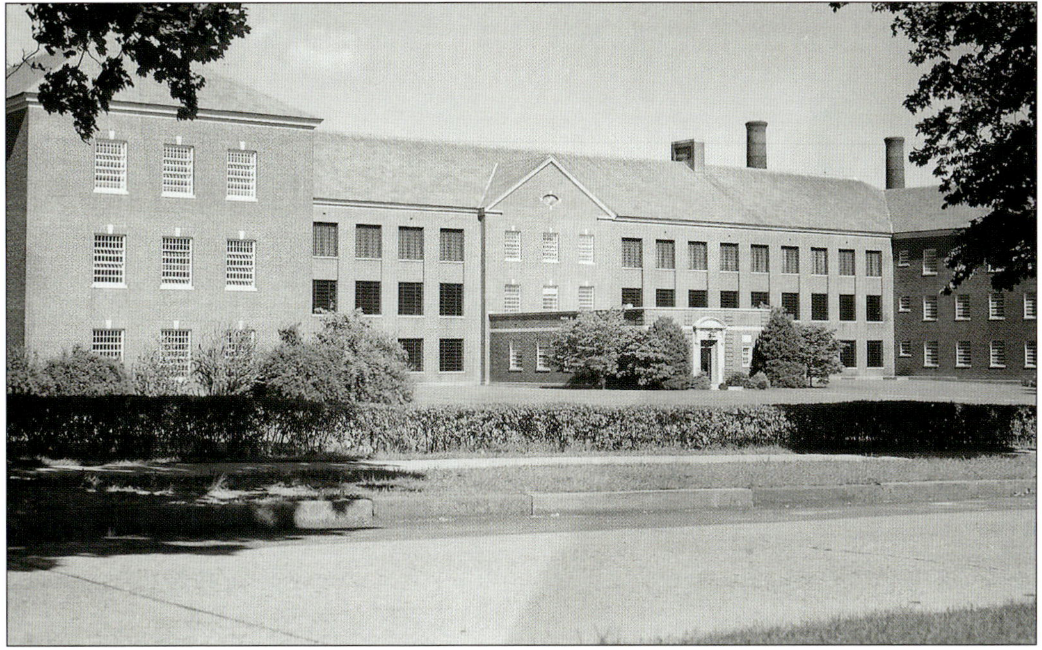

Sam explained that his hesitation, and even fear, came from the unknown. Since he was young, his friends teased him when they found out he was going to work at the center. They filled him with fear of the imagined nightmares he would face. (Courtesy of the Leo P. Ostebo Kings Park Heritage Museum.)

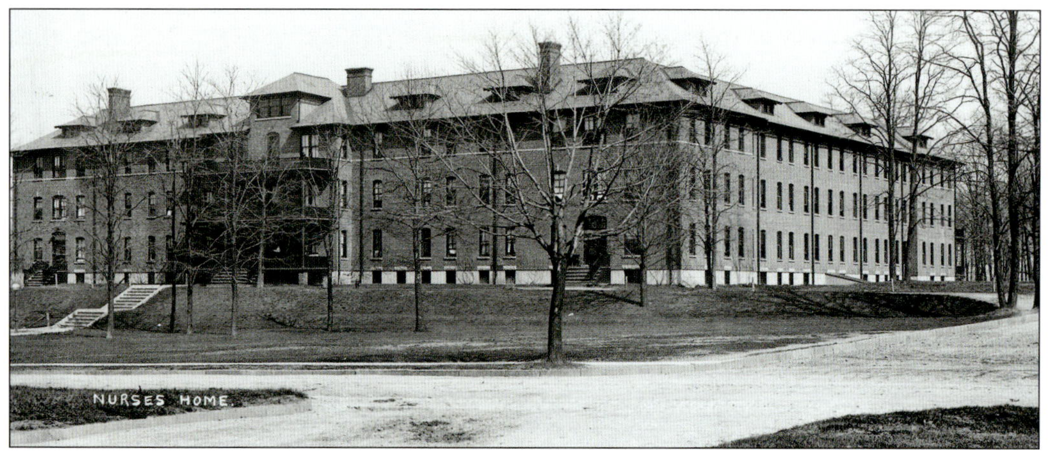

Shown here is the nurses' home. Sam contemplated not going in, quitting before he began, but as he said: "In those days, you make a commitment, you follow through. It was a matter of honor, of pride." Taking a deep breath, he threw open the doors and walked in. (Courtesy of the Leo P. Ostebo Kings Park Heritage Museum.)

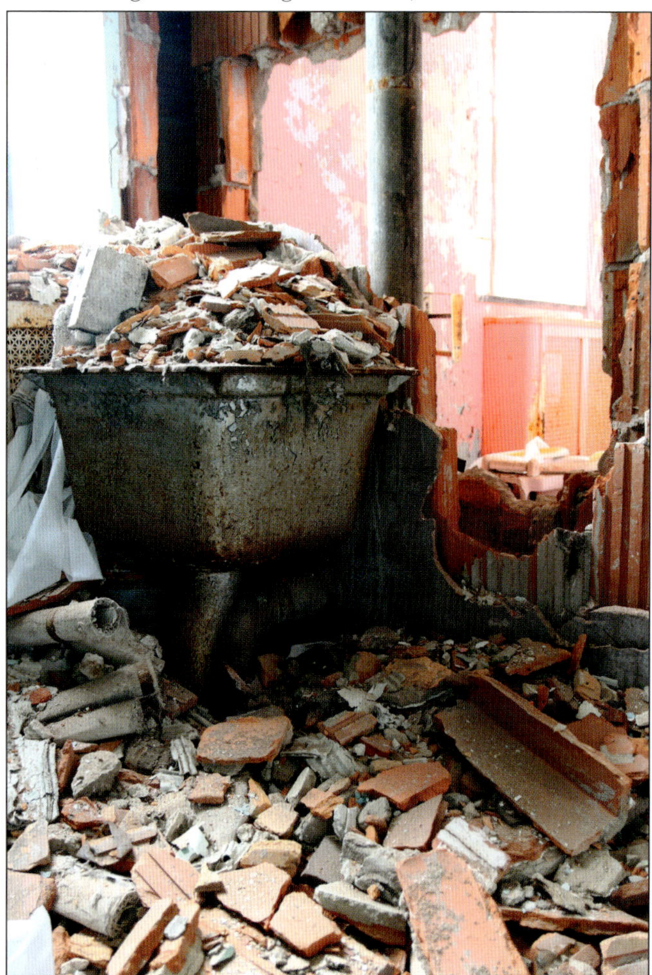

As soon as he entered, Sam was handed keys to the ward he would be working. His first duty was to assist moving the men from his ward to the dining hall. He was directed to a few male patients who needed assistance eating. His freshly pressed, pristine white uniform didn't remain so for long. Only a few minutes into the meal, Sam was wearing much of it.

Sam laughed remembering this first day. He said it was his own fault. The patient had told him he was done. By the end of the day, he said he was exhausted from a hard day's work, but he already loved it. After graduating high school, he had left for several years to serve in the Army. He saw the effect war had on his fellow soldiers.

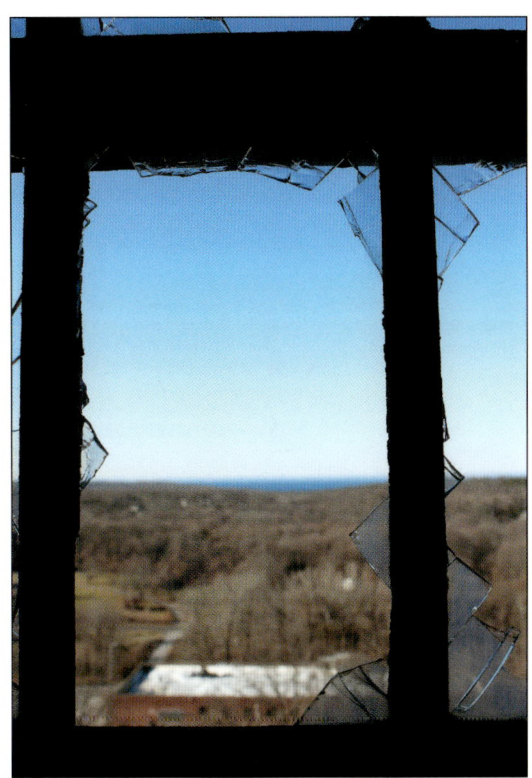

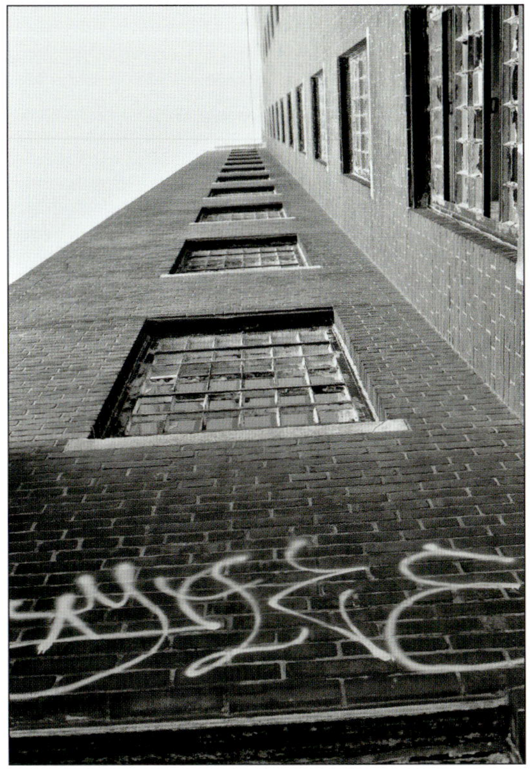

Once he finished his time in the Army, Sam returned to Kings Park, and immediately reapplied to the Psych Center. He was soon rehired and fell right back into the routine of the facility. Sam took pride in the work he did. In those days, he worked as a page, which would be similar to an orderly in today's terms.

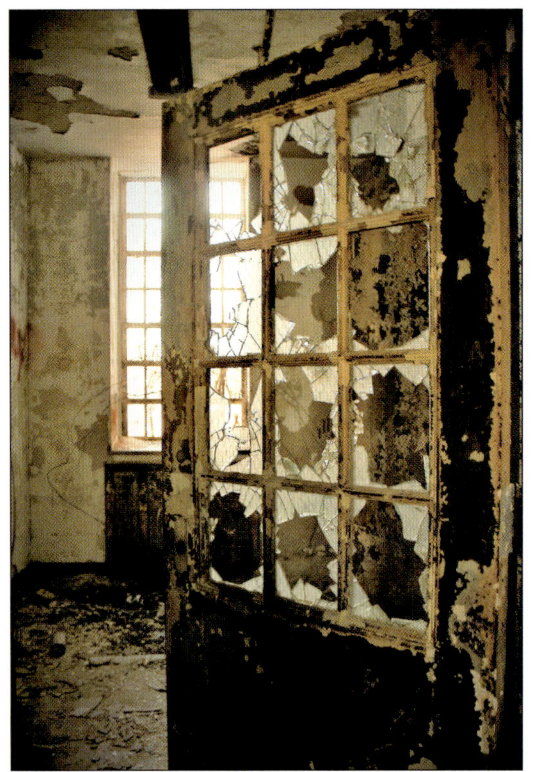

Sam smiled remembering his time at Kings Park: "It wasn't long after I came back that these patients began to feel more like family. A lot of these people had no one outside the center. Their families dropped them off and never returned. Not even after the patients had passed."

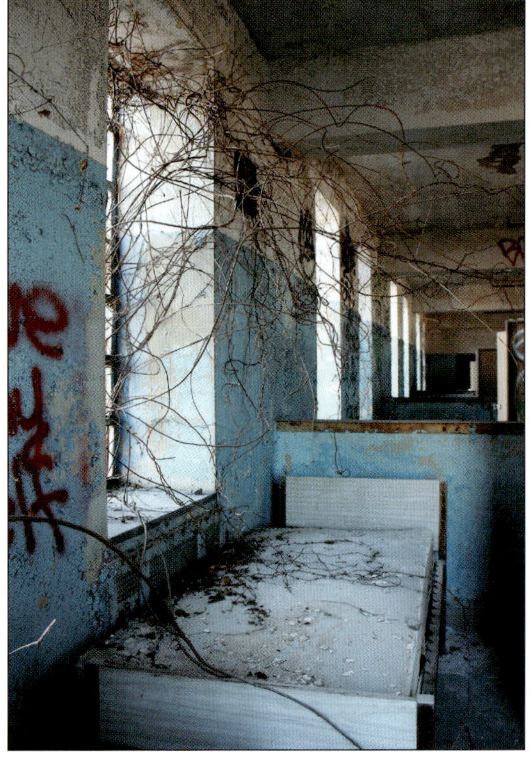

"But the people of the town, the employees too, would bring patients home for holidays. They just opened up their homes and welcomed them in." Sam paused, thinking back. "It's funny, thinking about my first impression walking in there as a kid. I was so scared, not knowing what I was walking into."

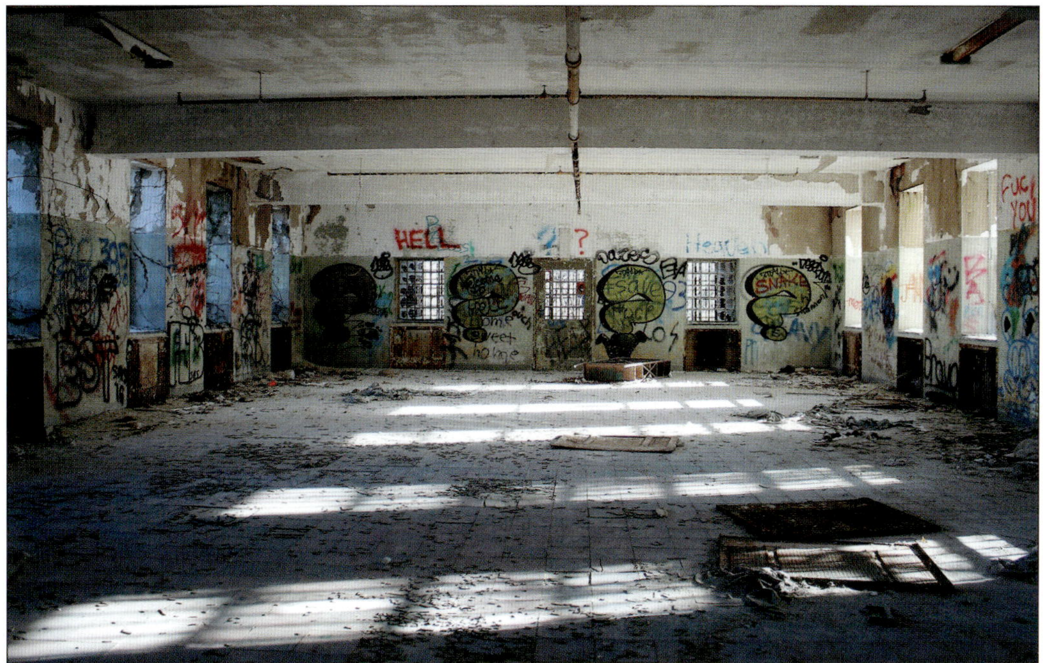

"Thinking back now. Now that I spent my life working in that place, I couldn't imagine my life without those people. Sure, there were times when it was scary. But the truth is, it was even more scary for the patients going through it. I was blessed to have been a part of it."

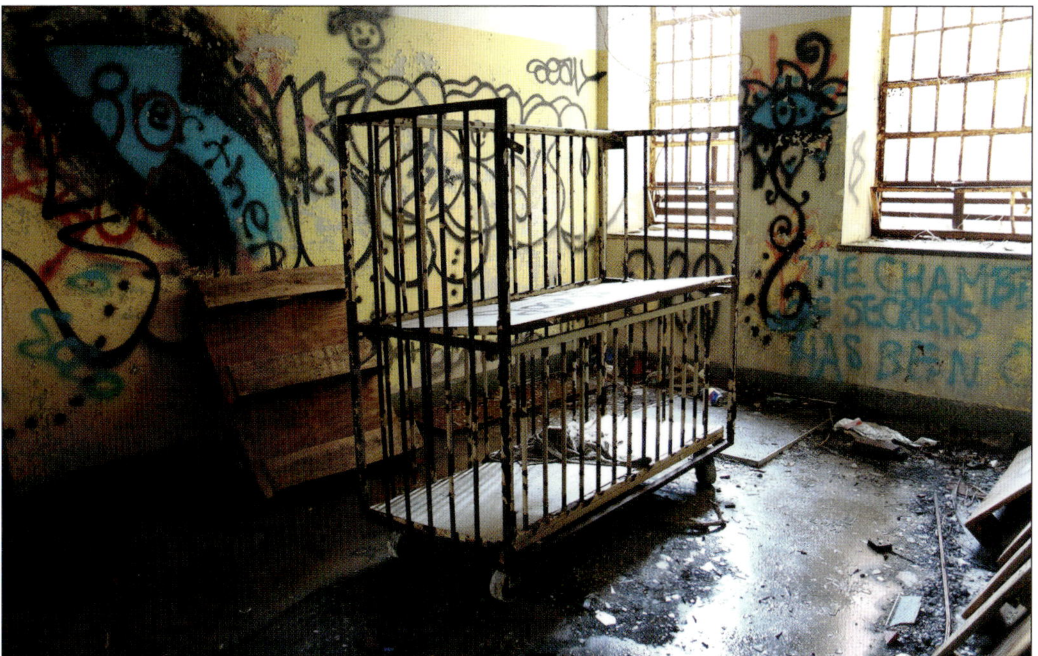

Kings Park Psychiatric Hospital, or the Psych Center, was noted as being on the cutting edge of psychological science. The center had earned a reputation for being an innovative facility, one whose caregivers would often look for new, and potentially better, techniques, procedures, treatments, and medications to better serve the population.

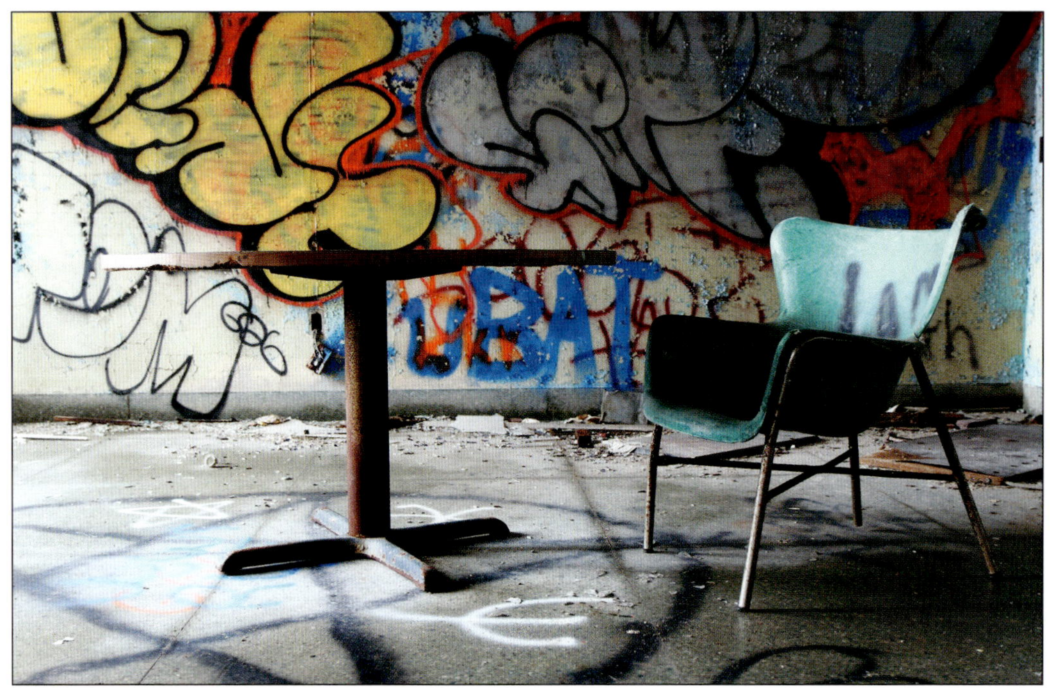

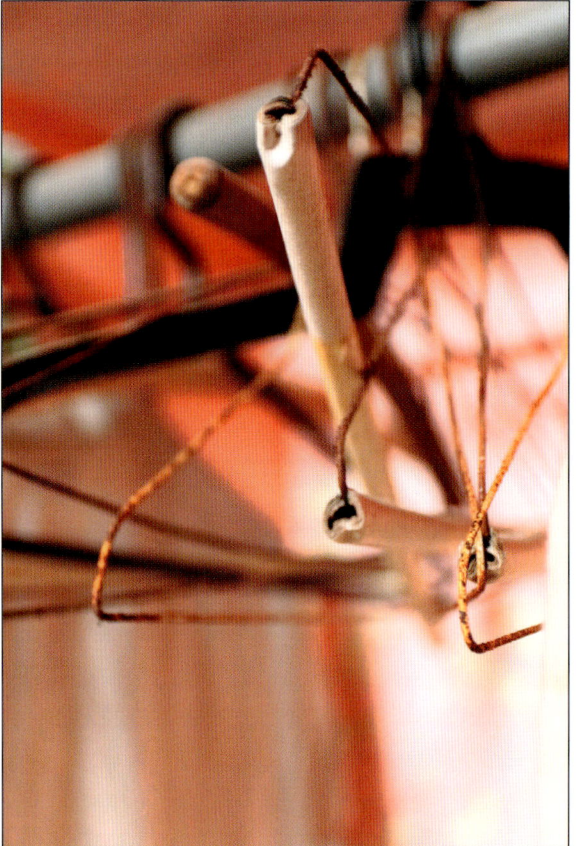

Prior to the advent of new treatment options, the psychological community, overwhelmed by the growing need for effective services, had reached a level of desperation. The overuse of restraints had become commonplace, and in much of the field throughout the country, employees were left to care for far too many patients, without adequate training and support.

In the 1940s, doctors in the psychiatric community began using shock therapy, also known as electroconvulsive therapy. It was felt that these treatments were an effective tool to help those patients with severe psychological disorders. Doctors, while working with patients with epilepsy, noticed that those with depressive symptoms seemed to improve after a seizure.

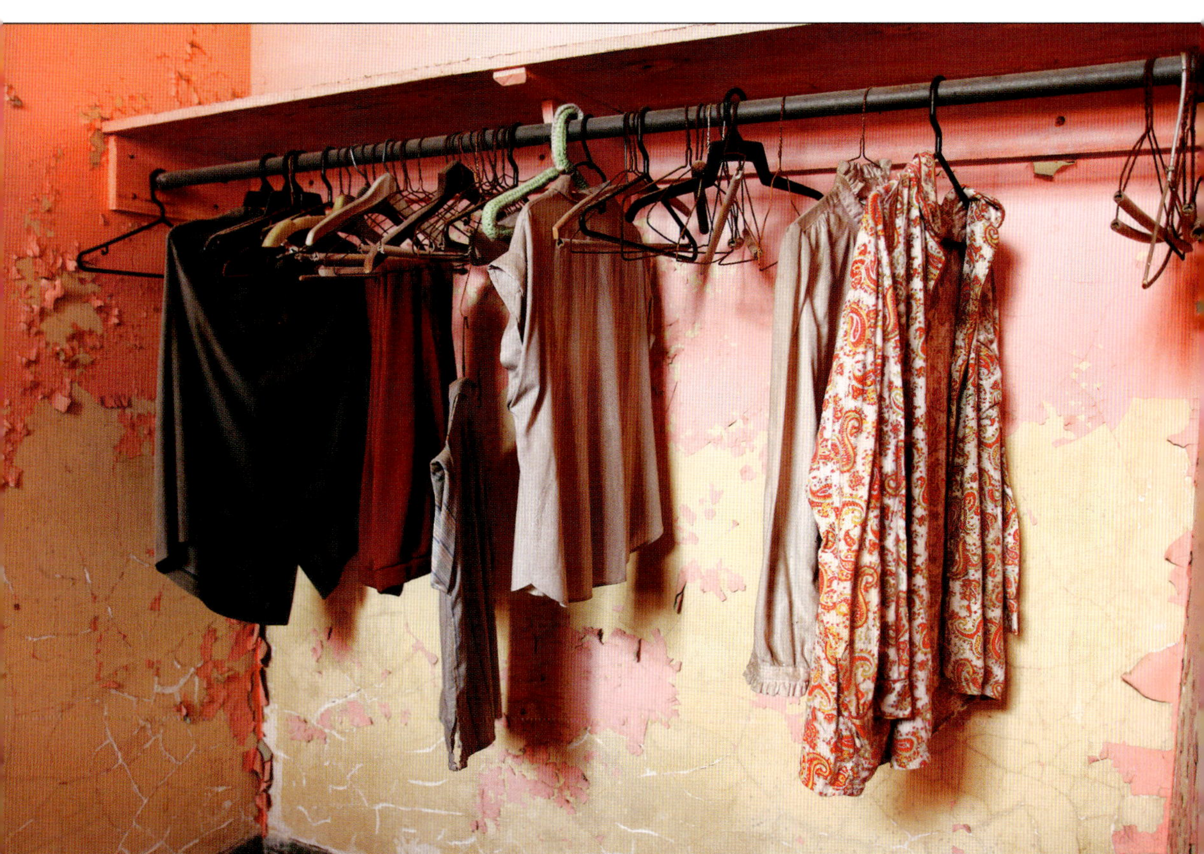

These "shock treatments" were intended to replicate the supposed benefits of seizures, but using electroconvulsive therapy (ECT) or insulin injections. A mild form of electroconvulsive therapy at a low sustained pulse is still used today in patients with severe symptoms that haven't been helped with other techniques, such as medication and/or talk therapy.

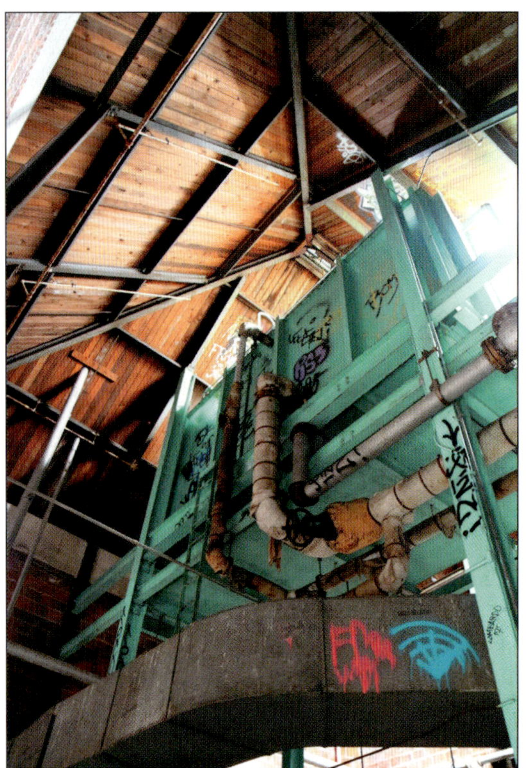

Electroconvulsive therapy is most commonly used in patients with severe major depression or bipolar disorder that has not responded to other treatments. Under general anesthesia, small electrical currents are passed through the brain.

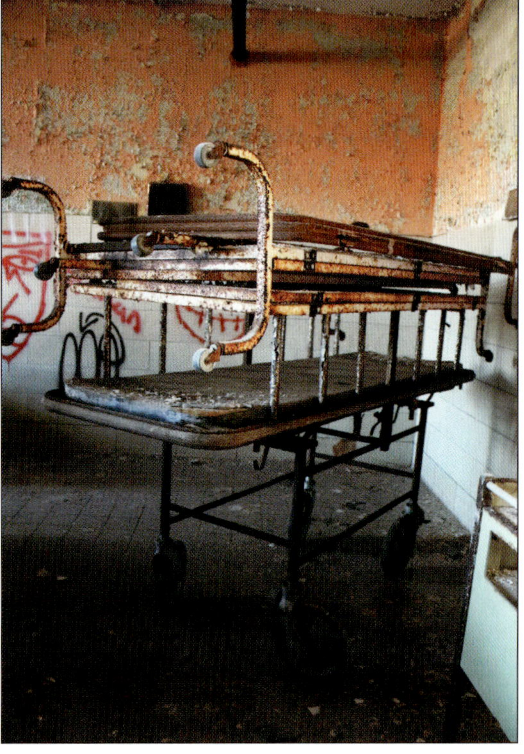

This is intended to cause a small, brief seizure, which appears to alter the brain chemistry and can reverse some symptoms of disorders such as major depressive disorder, bipolar disorder, suicidal ideations, and substance abuse, to name a few. Electroconvulsive therapy carried a horrifying stigma, based on a time when these treatments were given at high doses, often causing the patient undue pain, fractured bones and teeth, discomfort, memory loss, vomiting, and even death.

In some places, the patient would have been strapped fully conscious to a hospital bed and delivered the current at high voltage. Patients could convulse for up to 15 minutes at a time, causing damage to their bodies and minds.

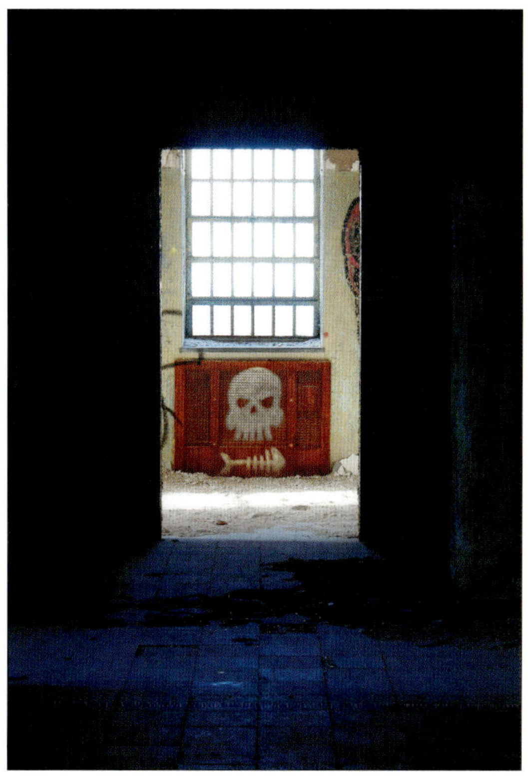

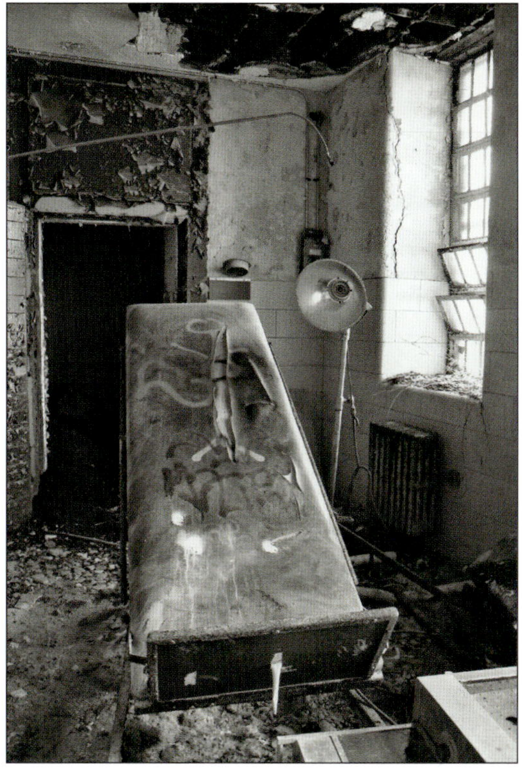

Unlike today, throughout the country, patients were not given the opportunity or even right to refuse treatments. Once a patient was admitted to an asylum, he or she had no right to give or deny consent for these procedures. In many cases, shock therapy was used as a punitive measure to keep unruly residents in line.

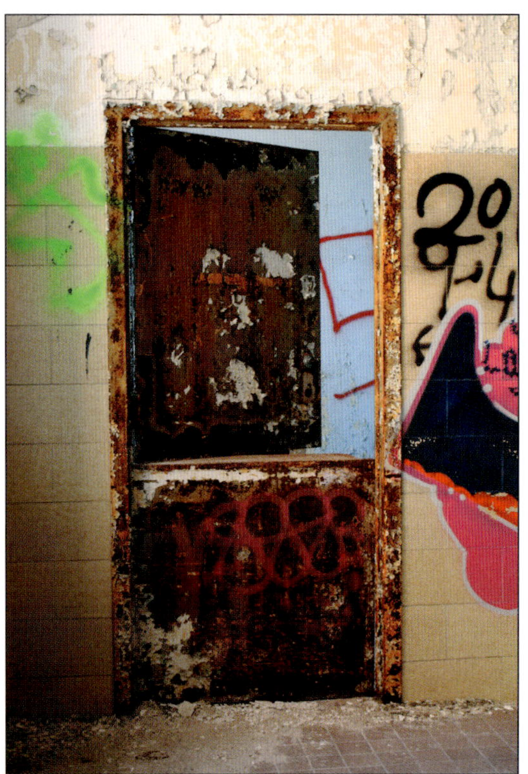

Long Island was made up of small villages, which made up the towns known today. Smithtown was well established as a shipping and milling community. Being perched at the point where the Nissequogue River was no longer navigable made it a prime location for this activity. These photographs were taken on the Mental Retardation Unit.

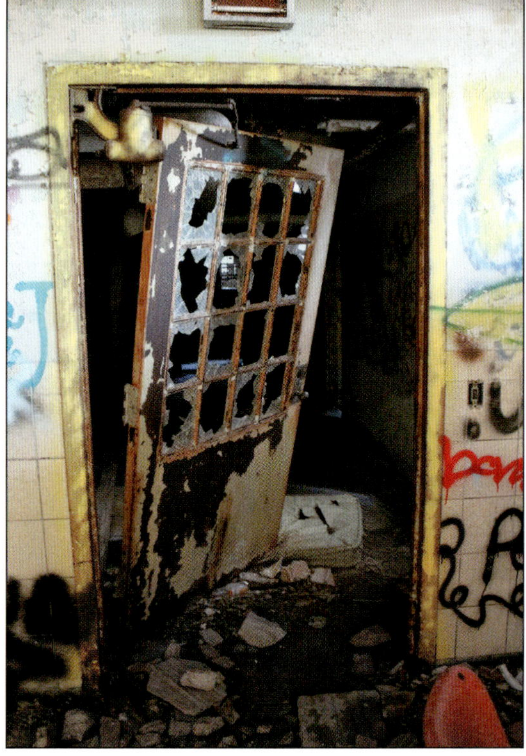

Northport, a historic maritime village, had been purchased from the Matinnecock Indian chief Asharaken for two coats, four shirts, seven quarts of liquor, and eleven ounces of "pawther" on October 15, 1656. Northport is in the town of Huntington on Long Island. Originally called Great Cow Harbor by 17th-century English colonists, it was officially renamed Northport in 1837. It was later incorporated as a village as part of an effort to organize a local government in 1898.

Now coterminous with the borough of Brooklyn, Kings County had established a "lunatic asylum" in 1829. This facility began with just seven patients living in a temporary building. By 1832, a larger, more permanent building was opened to accommodate the growing need for the care of patients.

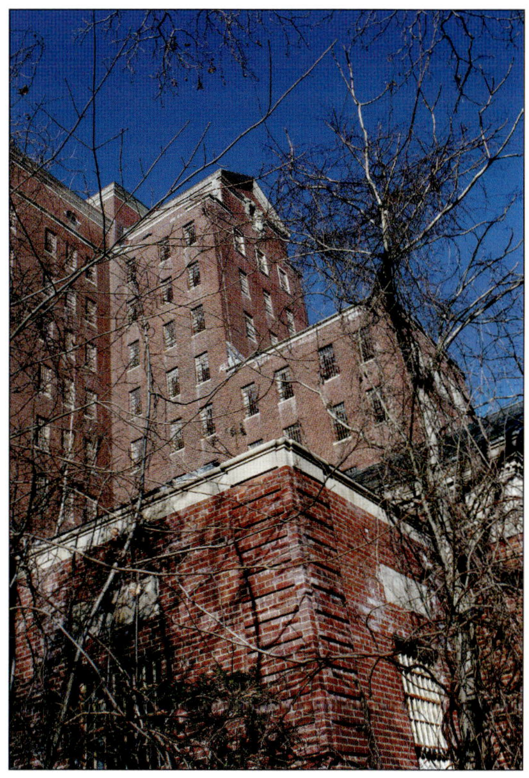

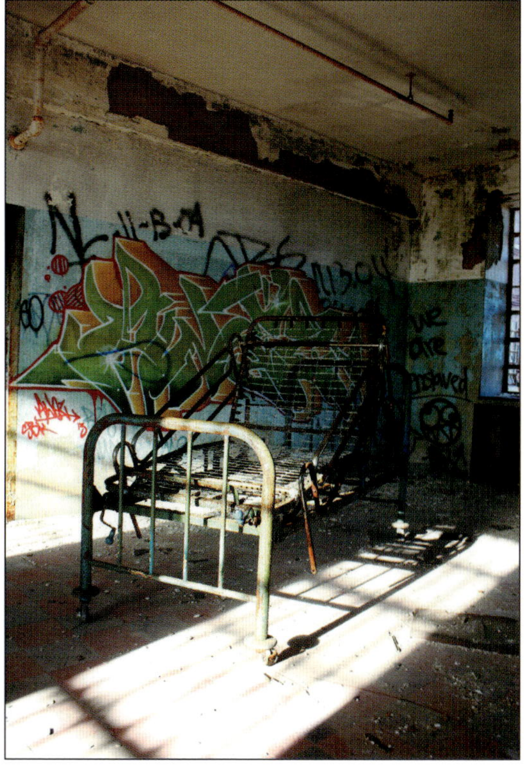

Over the next 50 years, the number of patients continued to increase, and the facility was struggling with overcrowding, as many other similar facilities were across the country. In one building that was designed to hold 600 patients, the number had grown to over 800.

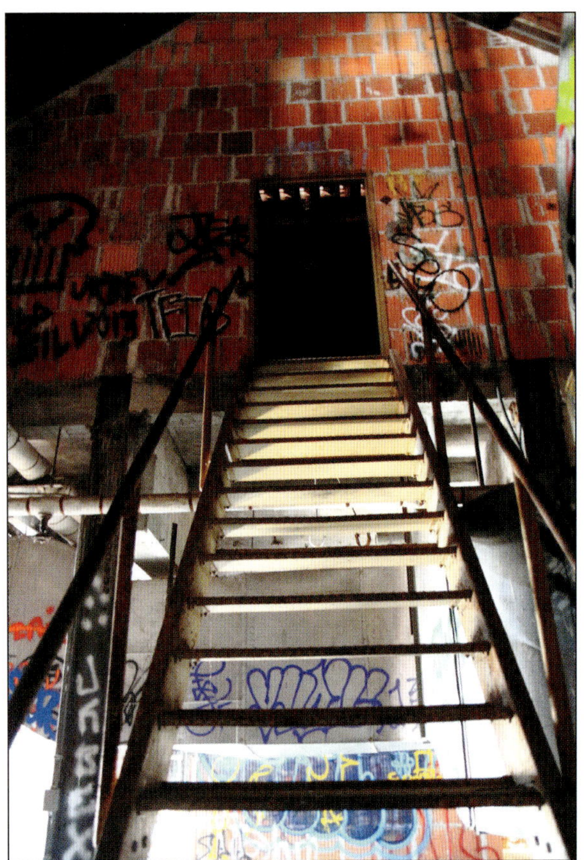

In 1866, Rev. William Muhlenberg, who also founded St. Luke's Hospital, took on another venture. In the town that is now known as Kings Park, he opened an orphanage and poor farm. This new venture was supported by donations from several wealthy families who had summer homes on Long Island. They purchased 400 acres of farmland in Smithtown.

Reverend Muhlenberg was deeply disturbed by the growing number of homeless in New York City, and organized his wealthy friends, and their contributions, to open the orphanage and poor farm. He conceived a community that would provide a home for indigent men and orphaned children. His ultimate plan was for the homeless to be able to learn a trade and earn their way to a better life.

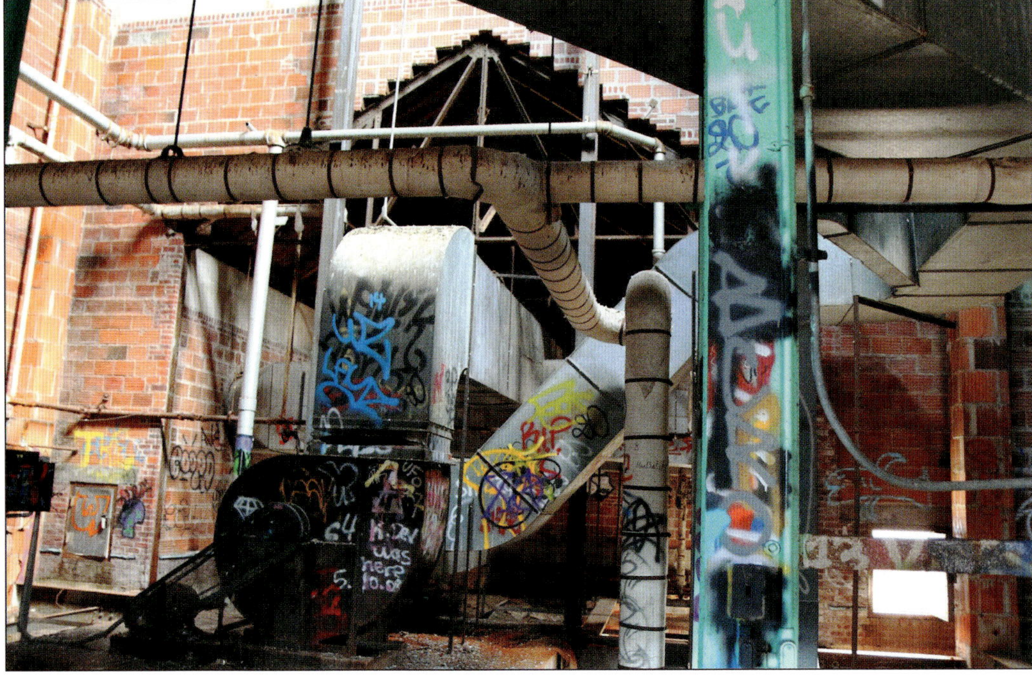

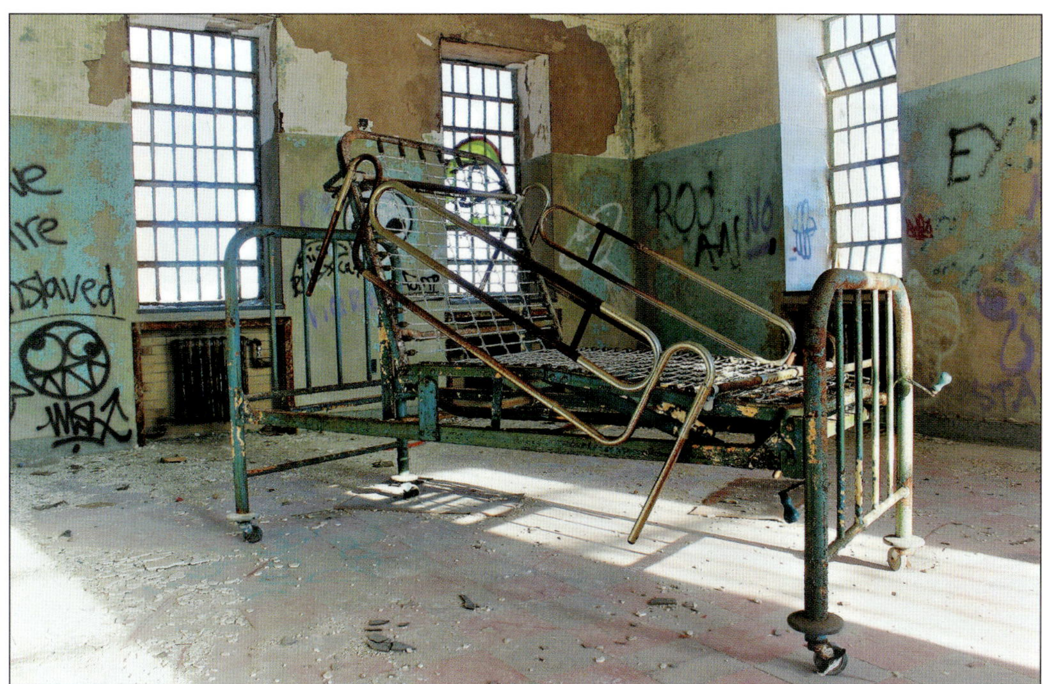

These homeless and the orphans could benefit one another and share the work, as well as a place they could call home. The homeless would farm their food and teach the orphans. Muhlenberg saw this as a self-sustaining project. He named the community St. Johnland, and it soon became a thriving settlement that gave its name to a section of Smithtown and the nearby railroad station.

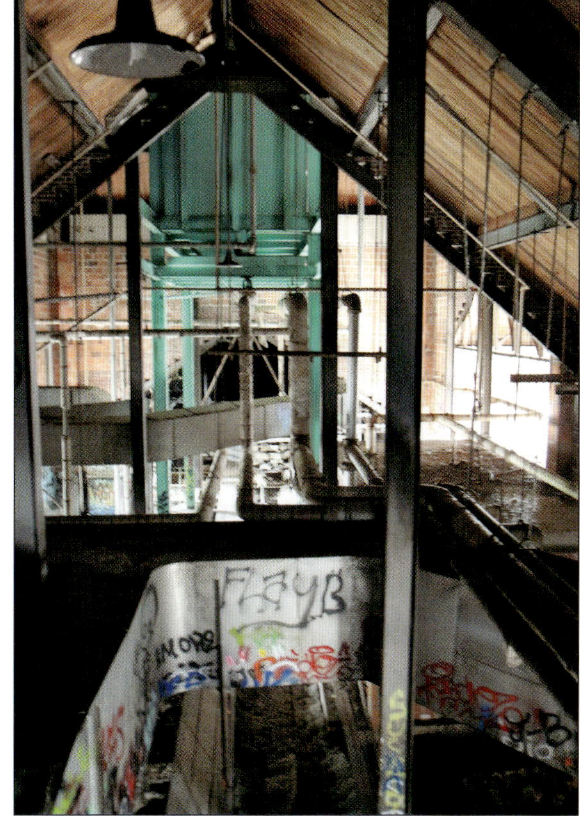

In 1865, in the first major change in the area, Dr. Oliver, a New York City minister, created the Society of St. Johnland, which purchased about 408 acres near Sunken Meadow Creek to build a community for orphans, the poor, and the elderly.

Kings County was becoming more heavily populated. After the new facility was established, and later occupied in April 1832, a small building had just seven living there. Over the next 50 years, the population of both the center and the community exploded.

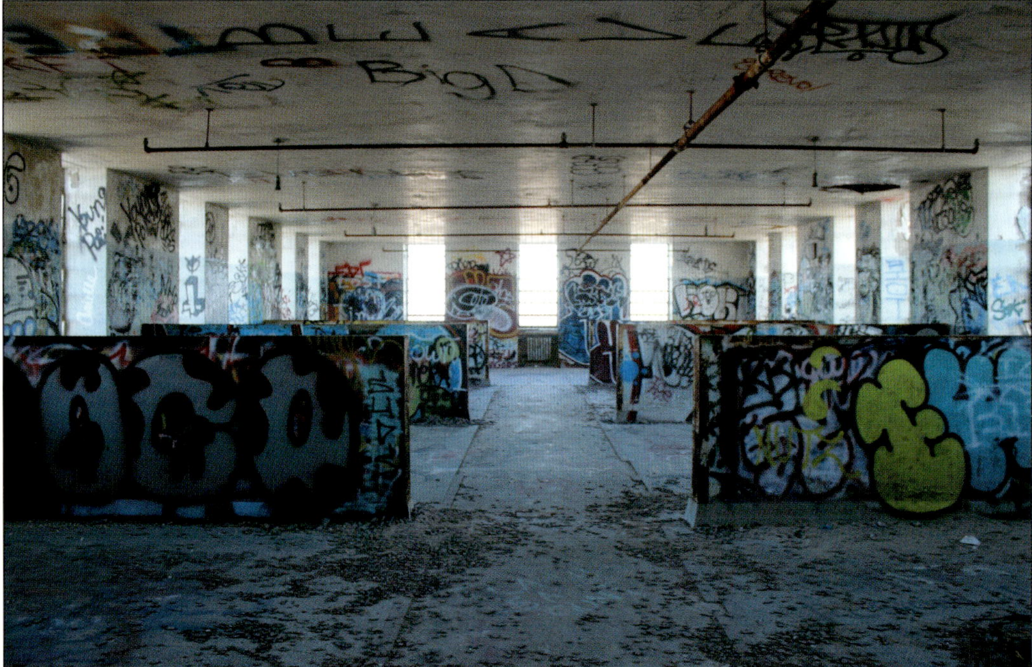

This rapid expansion of the population came partly from normal population growth and partly from the large influx of European immigrants. Unfortunately, many found it difficult to adjust to the new country, with a way life that was opposed to how they had envisioned it would be.

Though the county tried to keep up with the need for more beds by enlarging some of the old buildings and erecting new ones, the need grew faster, and there never seemed to be enough accommodations.

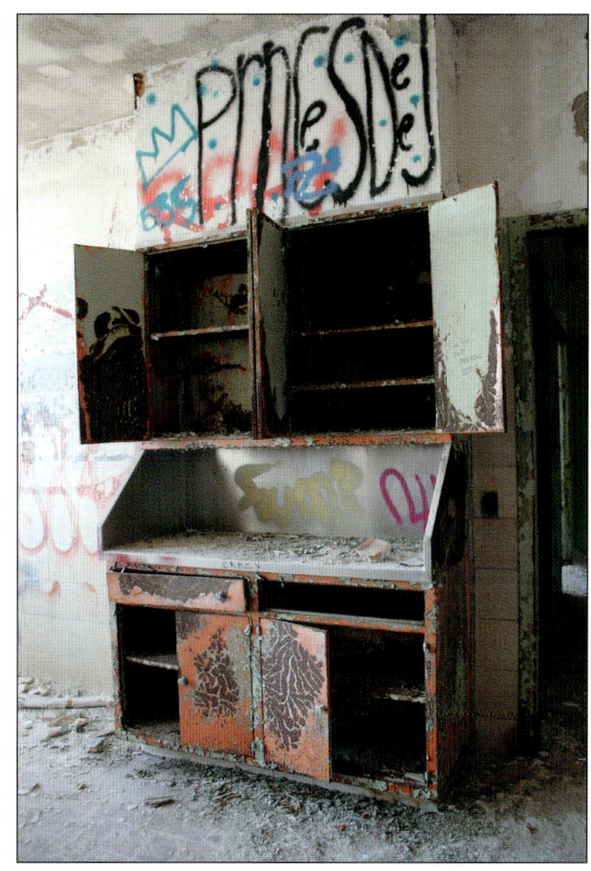

In 1871, a railroad company was incorporated to construct a line to extend the tracks from Northport, near what is now Stony Hollow Road, to Port Jefferson. A portion of this line would later be the route of Bread and Cheese Hollow Road when the line was relocated to make room for the iron trestle built over the hollow. On January 13, 1873, the first train came down this line from Port Jefferson.

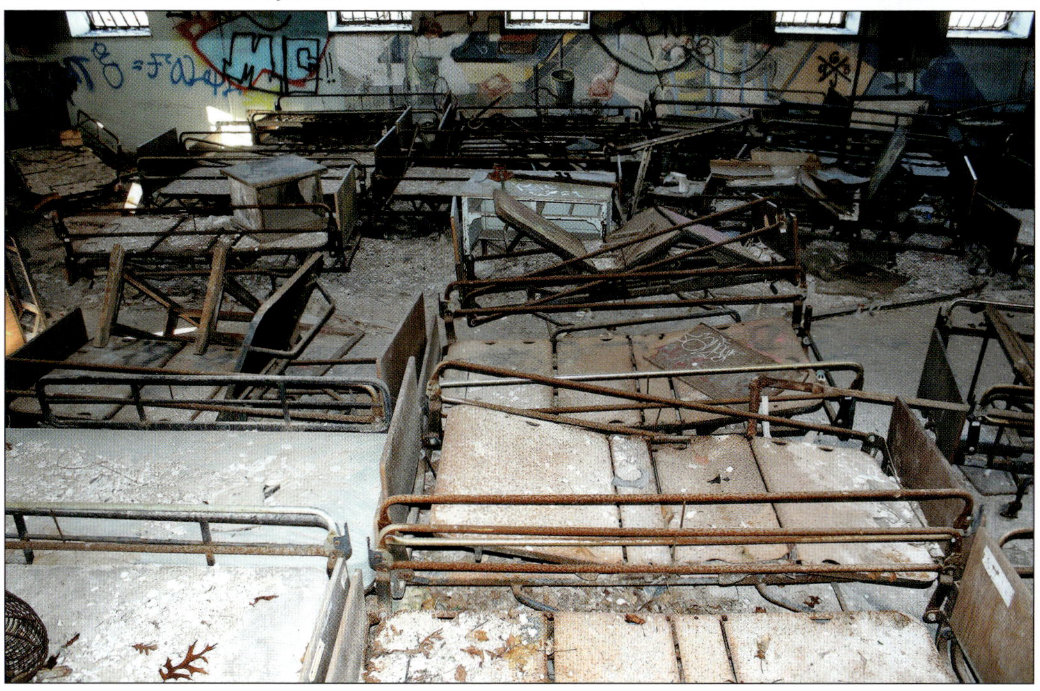

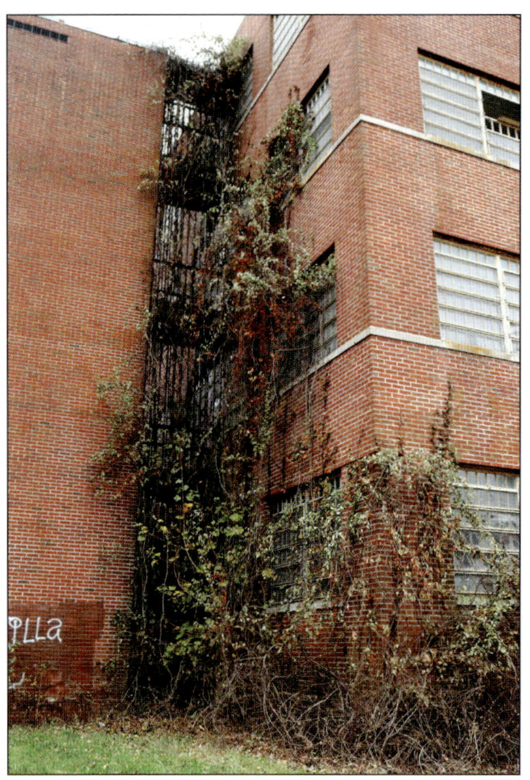

A new highway from St. John Road and the recently constructed railroad station was built in March 1873. The Town of Smithtown constructed this new highway, referred to as "the highway from head of the River to sunken Meadow." It was meant to make the railroad station more assessable. The new highway is now a segment of Route 25A.

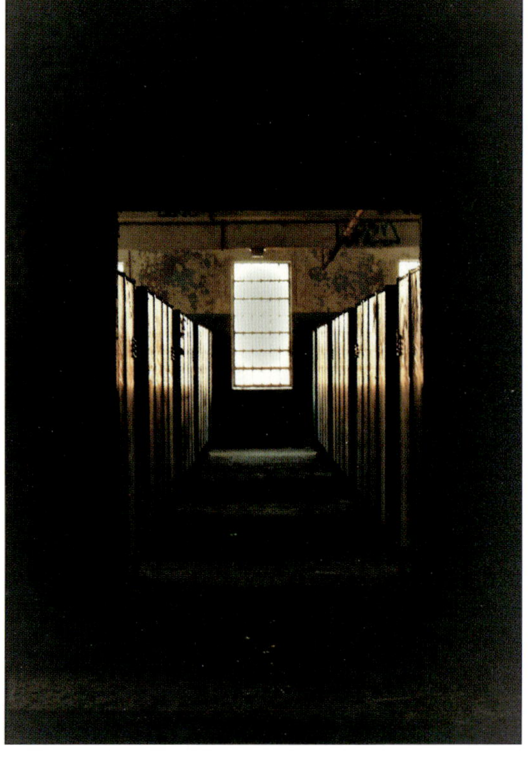

Excluding the seven buildings that were built in St. John, there were 15 houses built on the campus between 1858 and 1873, in what is now the hamlet of Kings Park. These additions brought the number of buildings to 78.

Two

The Late 1800s

The Kings Park State Hospital, as we called it, was where my father worked for 36 years. Almost all of his friends worked in the hospital, and it was the main employer of the town. The hospital was the main social conversation and entertainment entity in the town during the 1930s, 1940s, and 1950s. I was born in the 1930s, grew up in the 1930s and 1940s, and worked in the hospital in the 1950s. Because of this, I know how great an institution it was. Mainly, the reason was most of the people who worked there were warm, sensitive, sincere people who treated the patients as friends. My father brought patients home to have dinner in our house. During World War II, a patient was released to work at a war factory but needed a place to stay. He lived in our house until he got a place. In the 1930s, 1940s, and 1950s, the patients worked at many different jobs outside the ward during the day. They worked on the farms growing food, at the piggery, milking cows at the cow barn, helping the attendants clean the wards, etc. Most patients loved getting out of the wards and being productive; it made them feel good! Most of the hospital workers would buy patients candy, ice cream, cigarettes, whatever they liked, to reward them, to thank them; they did a good job! What made the KPSH a great hospital was the warm relationships between the patients and the hospital employees. The employees lived and believed in a certain way of life that gave them a certain type of compassion. If a patient needed something the hospital did not have, a lot of the workers would buy whatever was needed with their own money and bring it into work. The employees, who were mostly Irish immigrants, put on a St. Patrick's Irish Show each year for the patients and the town. The hospital had semipro baseball games at the hospital baseball field for the enjoyment of 500–800 patients three or four times a year. Many people in the town, including me, went to those games. Because of these memories and more, I can testify about the great care the patients got in the wards.

—Dr. George Tiernan
Kings Park Resident
Kings Park Hospital Staff
Kings Park Dentist

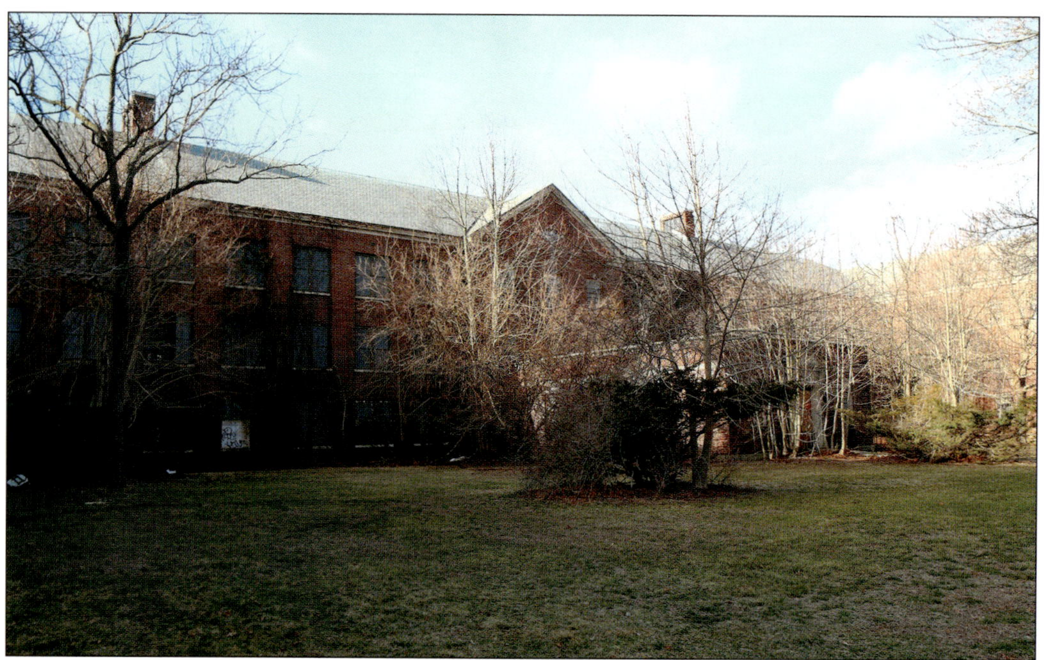

In 1879, the facility acquired a new superintendent, who was appalled by the living conditions of the patients and began to make changes. John C. Shaw, the medical superintendent, was horrified by overcrowding, the rampant use of restraints, and the dark, damp basement ward for females. The following photographs were taken on Wards 60–65.

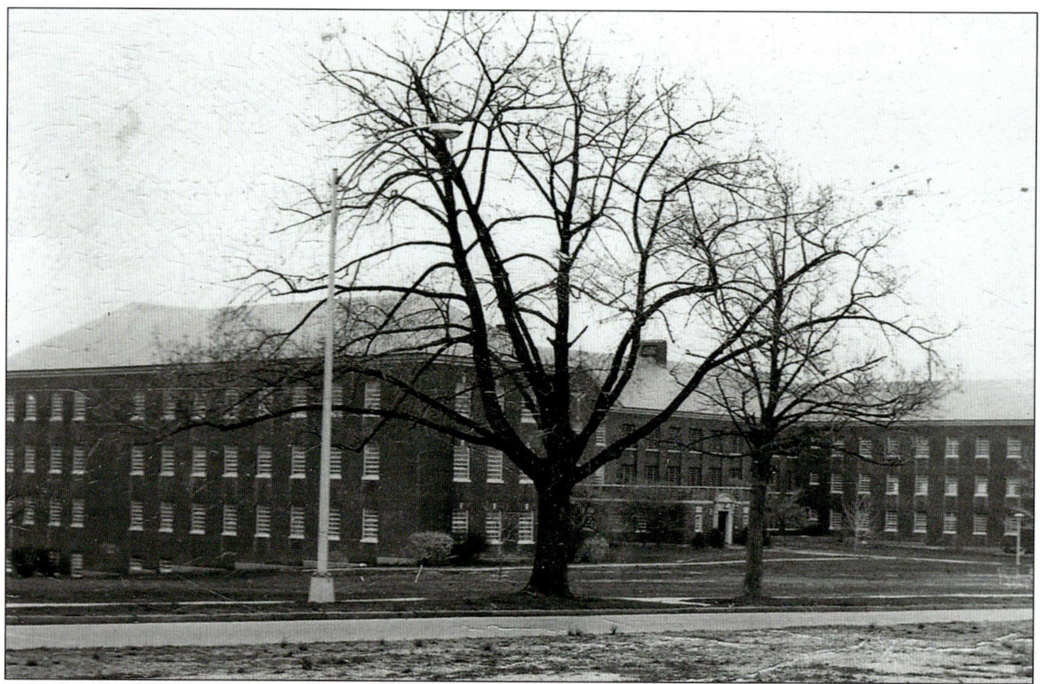

Superintendent Shaw began his advocacy for the patients. He felt they should have a more homelike environment, and the hospital should create a rural village setting. He knew that this would be the only home some of the patients would know.

Shaw felt an environment such as this would be more conducive to the morale and health of the patients. He suggested and pushed for a change in the method of caring for the insane. He felt that the asylum should be moved into a suitable and healthy location. The campus, he proposed, could be developed with "detached buildings of various sizes . . . built so as to have a small village."

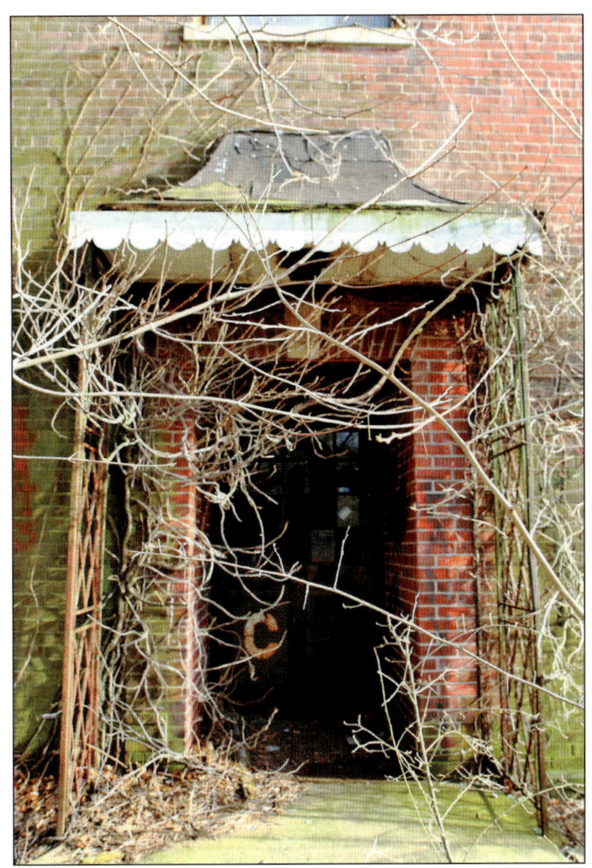

This would provide homelike surroundings, plenty of room, occupations, and a more natural life to the chronic cases, and immensely improve the chances of recovery for many. In 1880, the Edward Thompson publishing company was created with the purpose of publishing an encyclopedia of law. It was so successful that by 1887, the company erected a three-story brick building and hired 125 people. Most of those hired were young male attorneys who brought an atmosphere of culture and gentility to Northport.

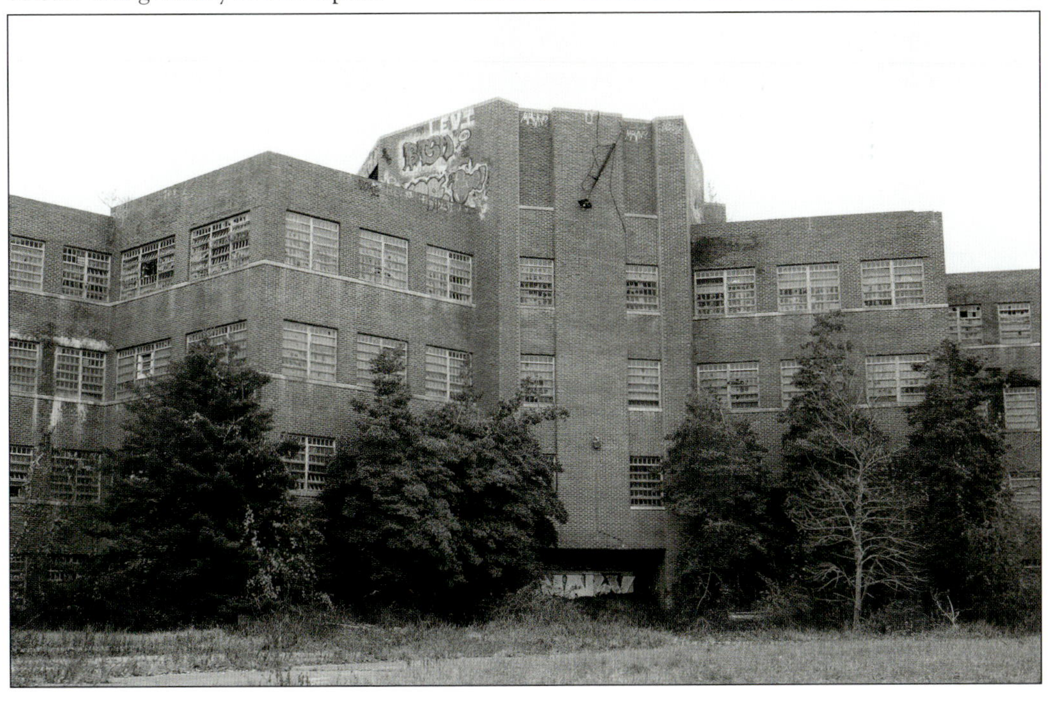

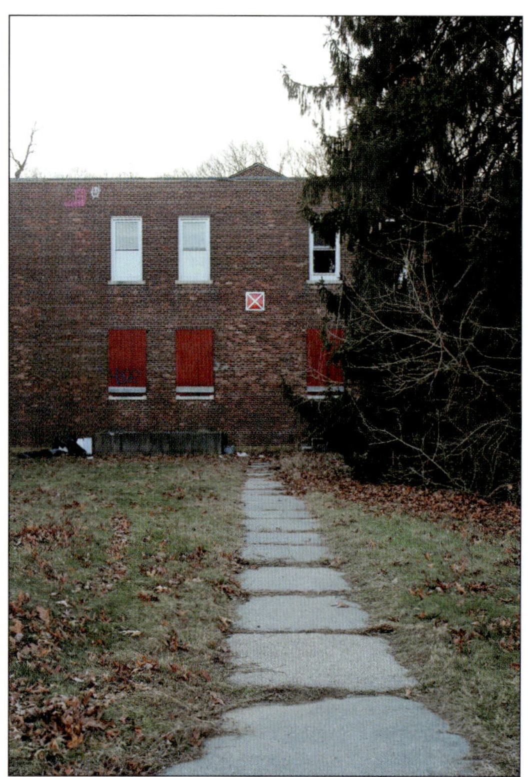

In 1885, Kings County purchased 875.8 acres of farmland near Muhlenberg's poorhouse and orphanage. In an area near the train station called St. Johnland, a new facility was erected and named St. Johnland Branch Asylum. Thirty-three male patients and 23 female patients were moved into the newly refurbished farm buildings. Conditions were less than ideal, some would even say primitive, and several patients ran away. This photograph was taken on Wards 90–100.

NOTICE
IN CASE OF FIRE FOLLOW
R-A-C-E
R - RESCUE- RESCUE ANYONE IN IMMEDIATE DANGER.
A - ALARM - PULL ALARM THEN CALL 2333 GIVING LOCATION OF FIRE.
C - CONFINE-CONFINE FIRE BY CLOSING ALL DOORS AND WINDOWS IN AREA.
E - EXTINGUISH-AFTER EVACUATING PATIENTS. EXTINGUISH FIRE.

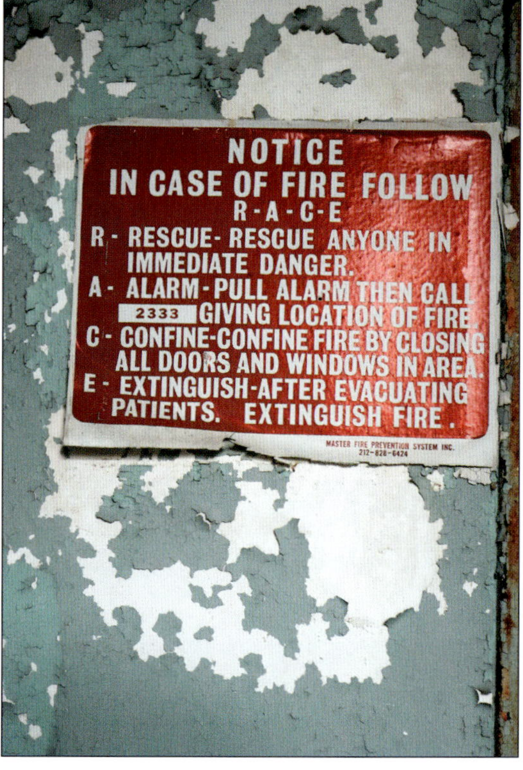

Sent by Dr. Shaw, an assistant physician was brought in to run St. Johnland. Prior to the consolidation of the five boroughs, the City of Brooklyn established Kings County Asylum in 1885. It was designed using the farm-colony model, which had become the popular style of the time. The following photographs were taken in the Medical/Surgery/X-Ray/Laboratory Building.

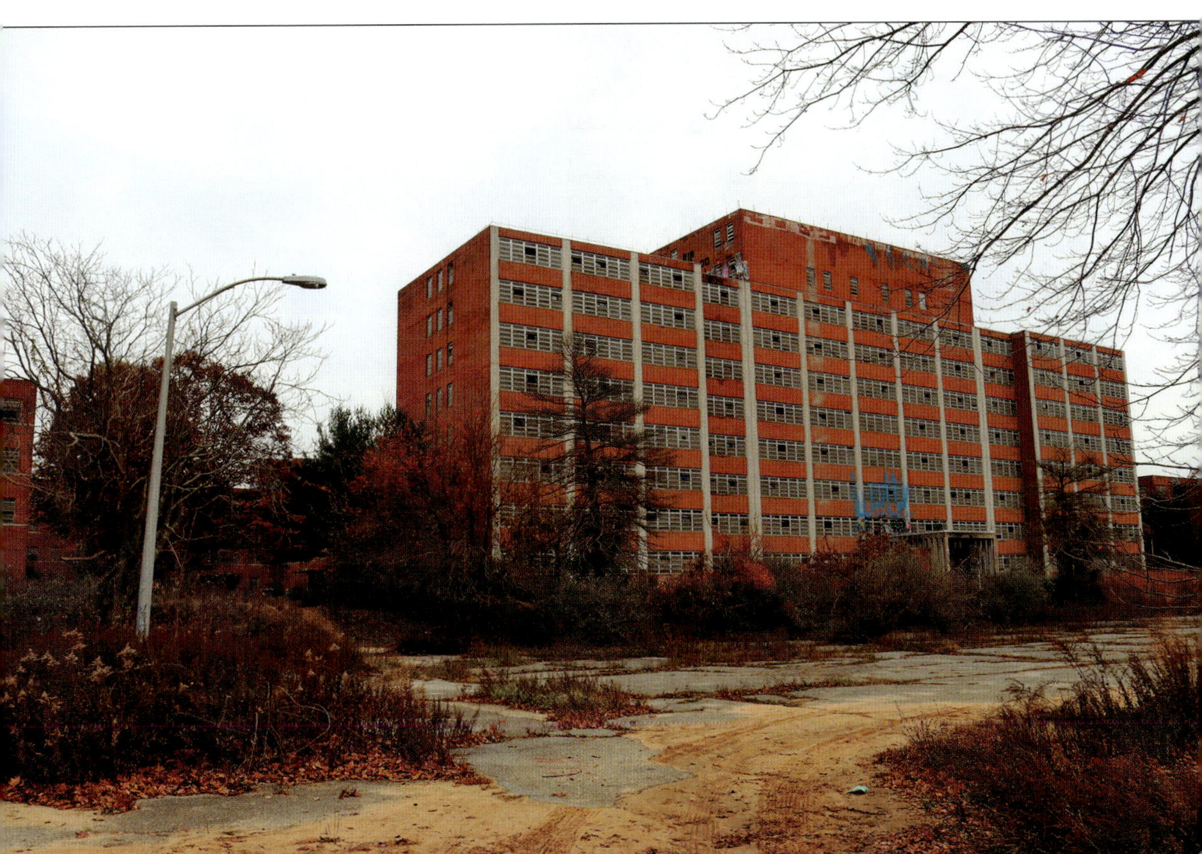

This type of campus was designed to be like a small town. It was a self-sufficient community where residents were put to work raising crops and livestock to support the sprawling campus. The labor was thought to be therapeutic, occupying the time and attention of residents and keeping costs down. It gave the patients a sense of purpose in addition to fresh air and sunshine.

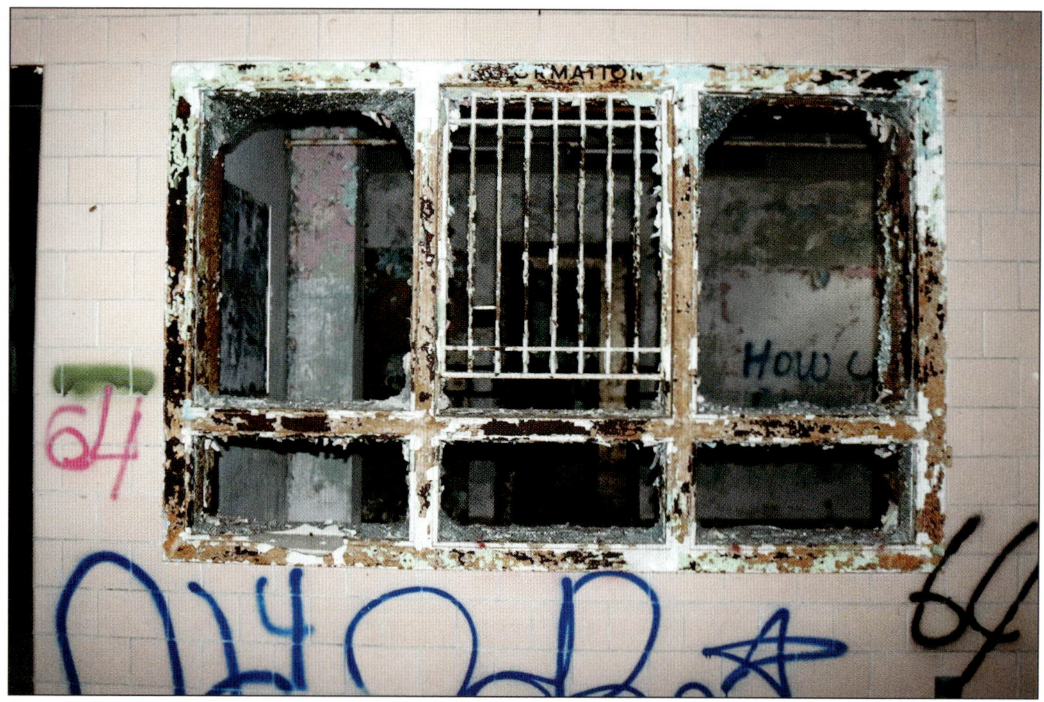

While this was but one of the three state hospitals built on Long Island in the 19th century, it opened its doors to curb the overcrowding at surrounding hospitals. Kings Park Lunatic Asylum opened in 1885 to an initial 55 patients.

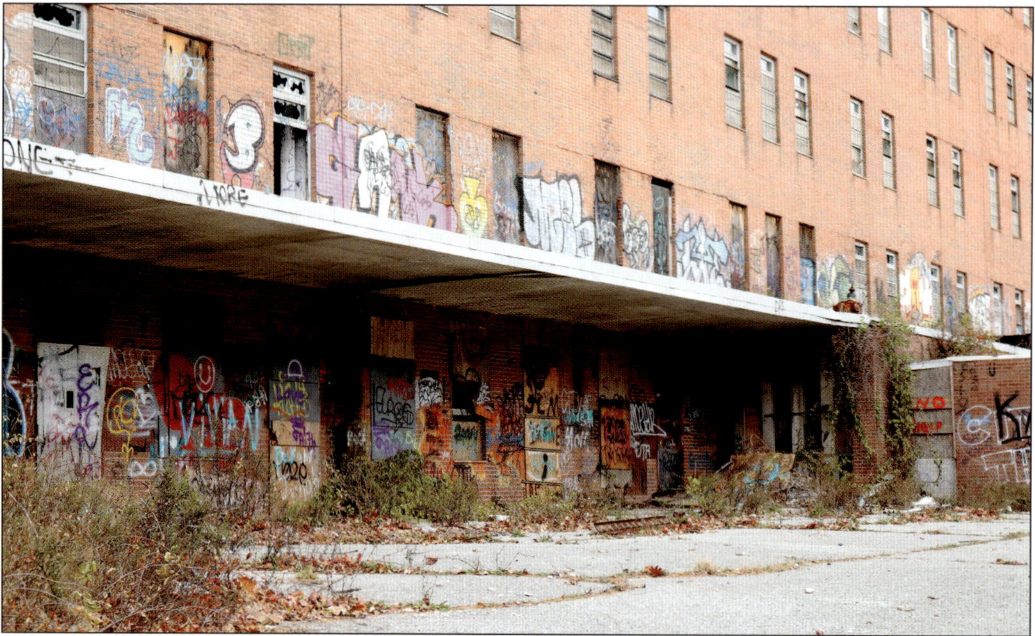

Ten years later, the State of New York took over the asylum after complaints of patronage and waste of resources that arose from both the asylum's staff and the general public. It was at that time that the name was changed to Kings Park State Hospital. The whole site is now known colloquially as the Kings Park Psychiatric Center, or KPPC.

By 1887, three new temporary buildings had been built, and 200 patients were moved into them from the Kings County Asylum. Two years later, with the relentless need for more beds, more cottages were built, along with a laundry, heating plant, barns, and more.

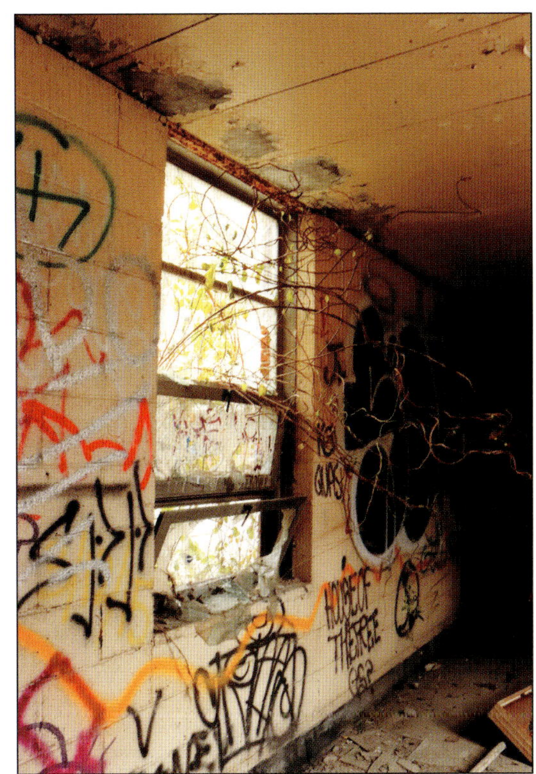

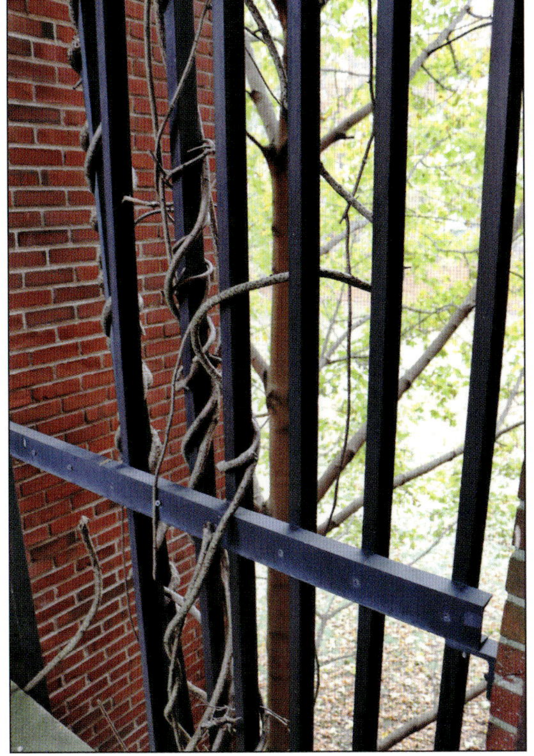

Hospital administrators were able to add 450 patients to the campus. Three temporary buildings were erected in the fall of 1887, and 200 patients were sent out. This established a pattern of building to meet expanding needs that was to continue for many years.

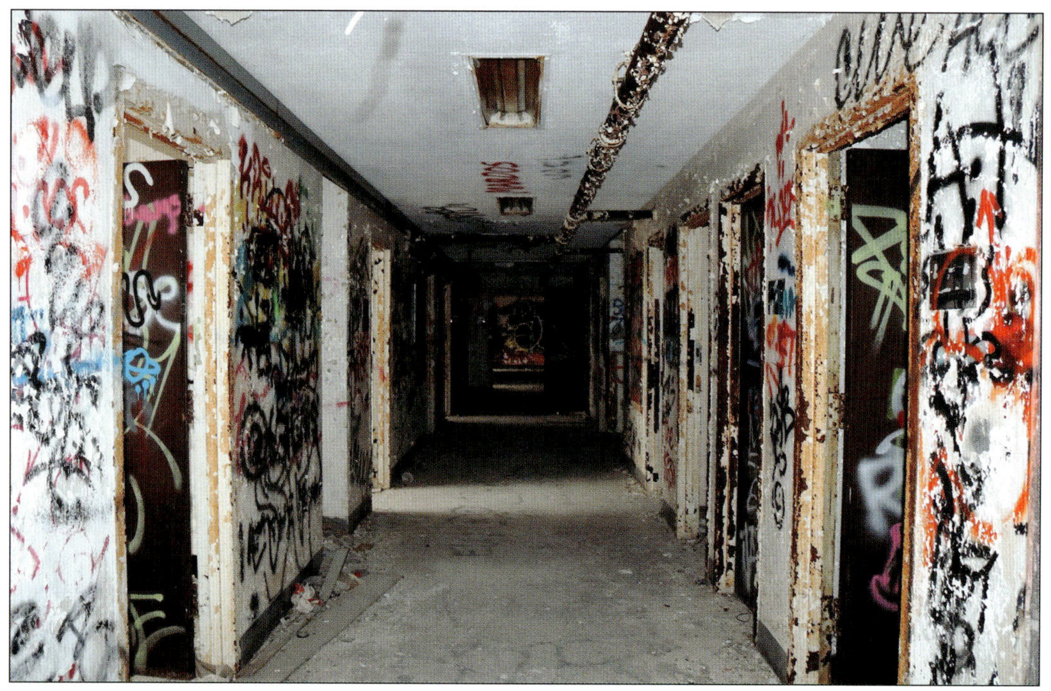

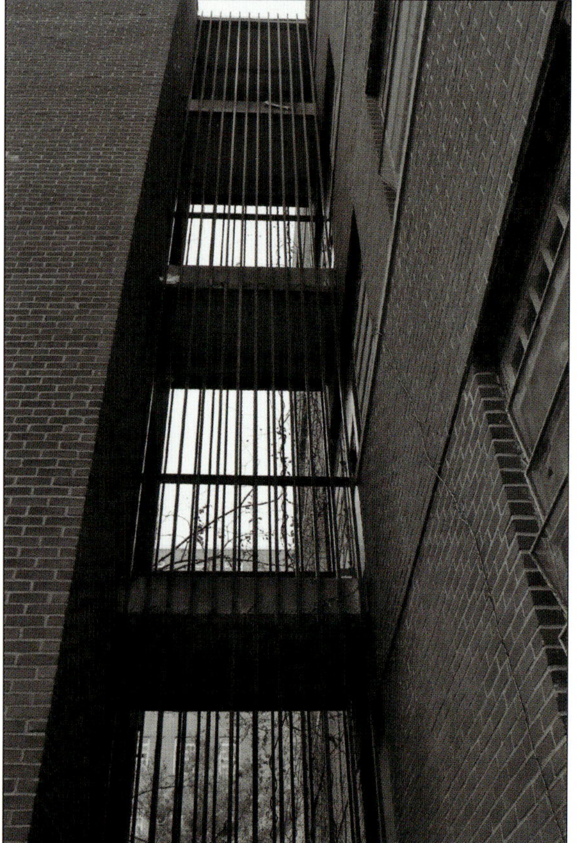

Benjamin Gay became president of the commission of charities and corrections of Kings County in 1889. Serving with him were George H. Murphy and Francis Nolan. They were not known for their compassion for the mentally ill or for their care. Shown here is Building F.

While construction continued, it was later thought that these committeemen had only the intention to encourage considerable graft. While over 11 million bricks were used to fill in excavation prepared for the erection of a building, the huge number of bricks offered many opportunities for unscrupulous construction companies.

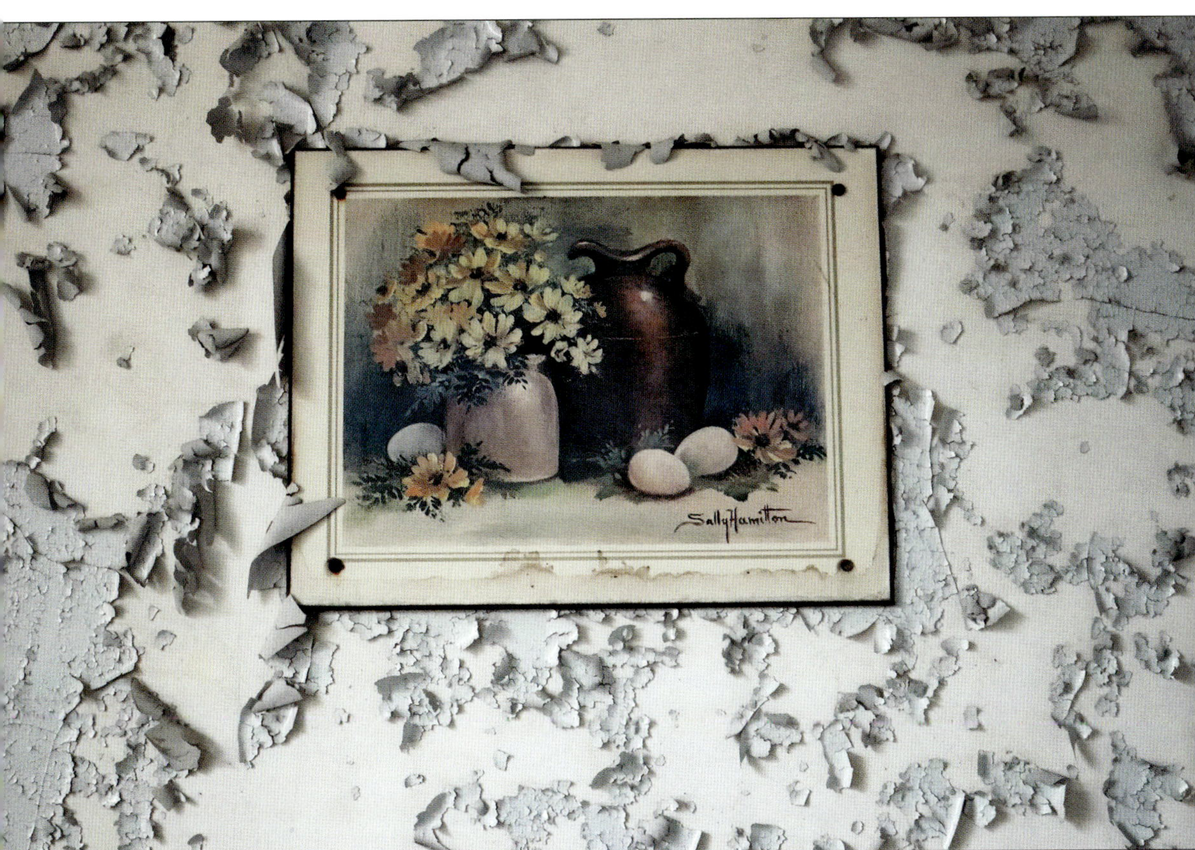

For example, one barge, loaded with barrels of cement for the construction site, sprang a leak that destroyed the entire shipment. However, the cement was paid for even though it was unusable. The following photographs were taken in the Medical/Surgery/X-Ray/Laboratory Building.

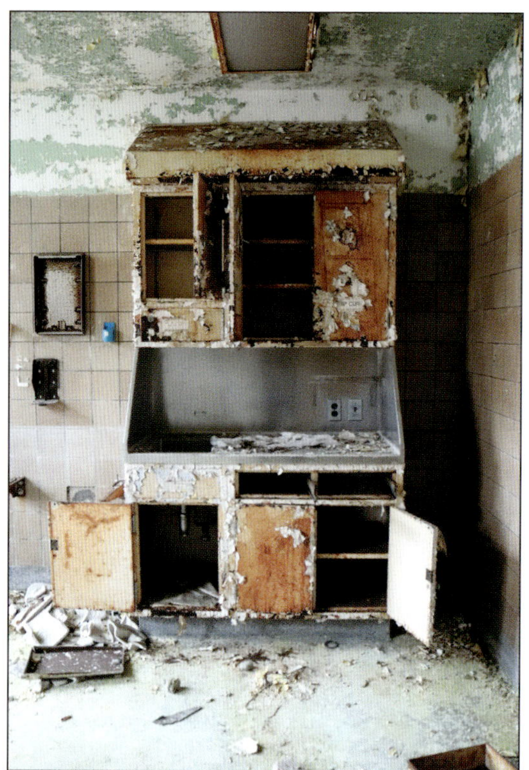

Hundreds of wagonloads of dirt were removed from the site chosen for reservoirs. The earth was carted a mile into the woods and dumped. Later, all the work was reversed as the same dirt was brought back to build embankments around the same reservoirs.

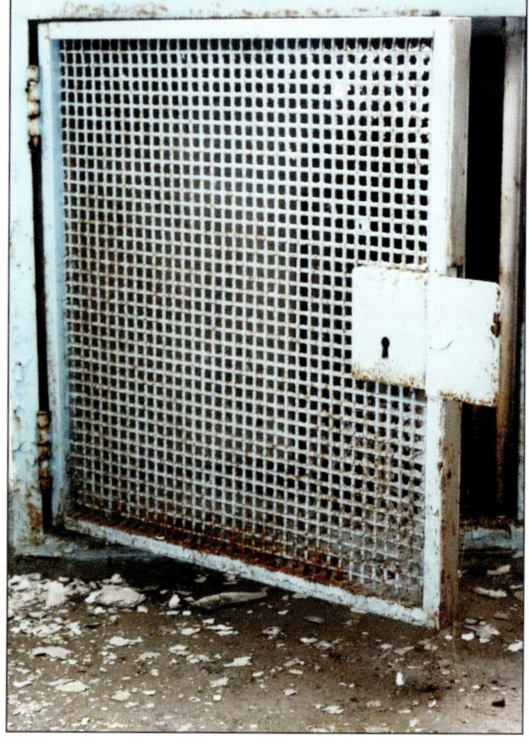

The railway station was originally known as St. Johnland. However, the townspeople objected to the idea that their train station and neighborhoods should share the same name as the asylum. In 1891, they changed the name of the station to Kings Park.

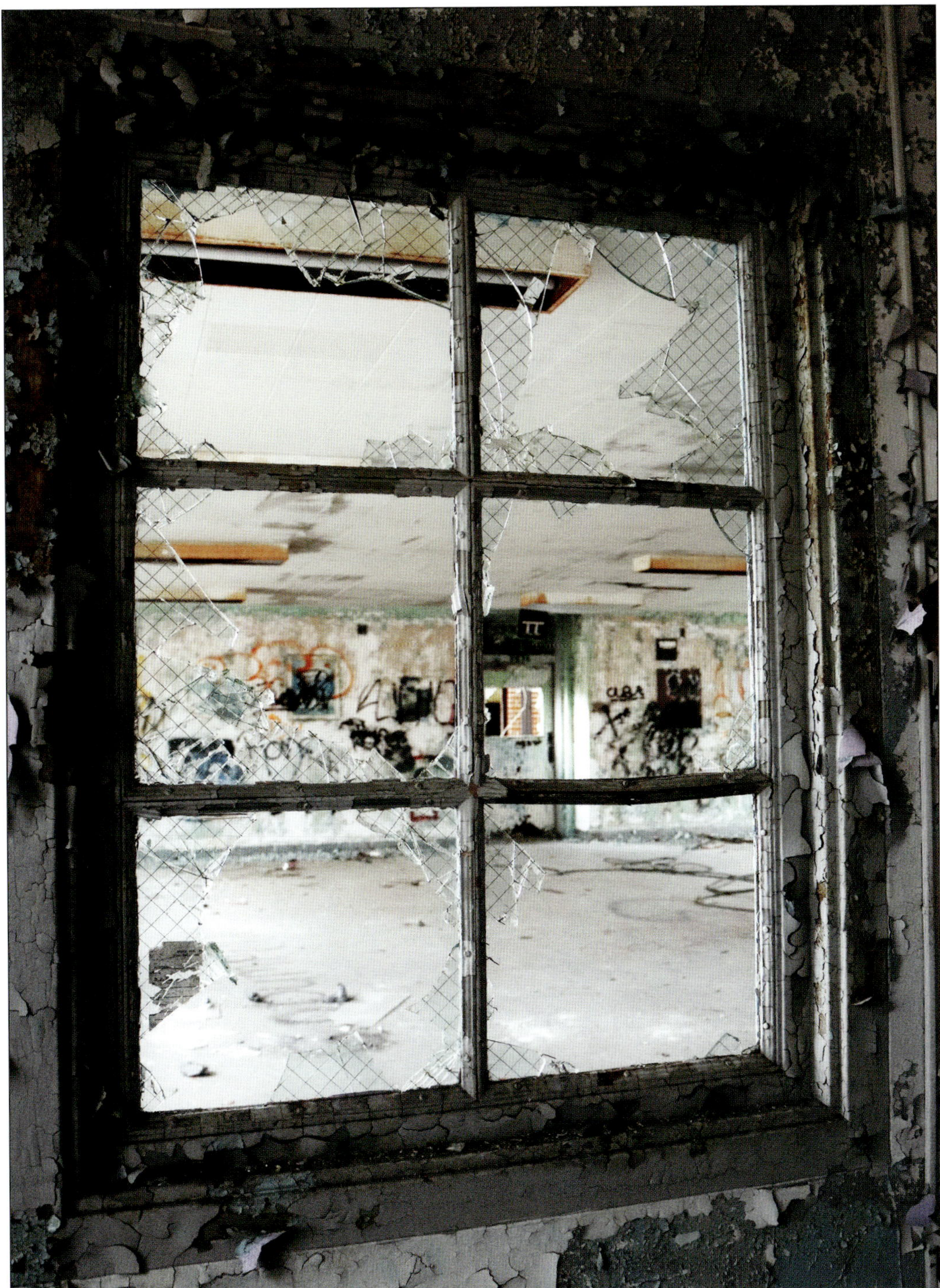

Kings Park Psychiatric Center, or the Psych Center, has also been called the Asylum, or the Kings County Branch Asylum. Former names of the hospital included St. Johnland Branch Asylum and Branch of Kings County Lunatic Asylum. With its change to becoming a state-managed facility, Kings County Asylum became the Long Island State Hospital.

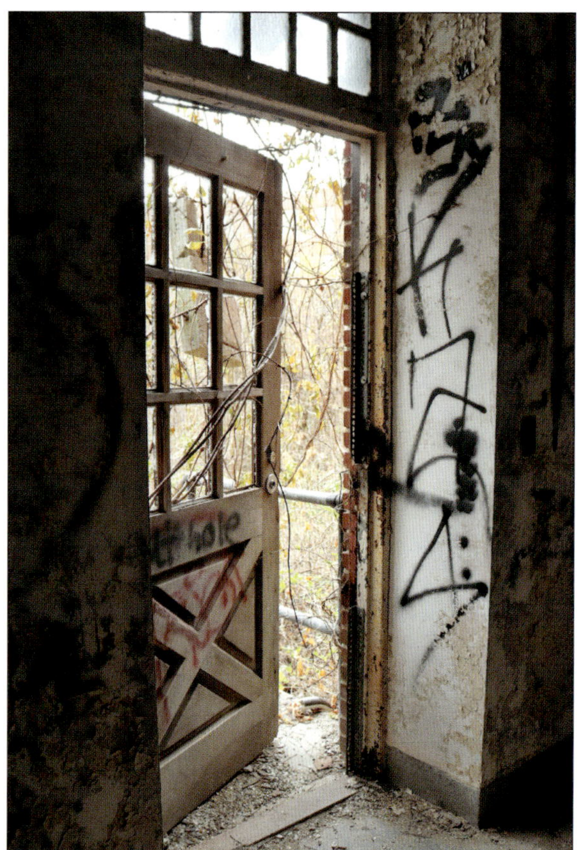

In 1892, the nurses and attendants began wearing more formal attire in the form of a uniform. Then, in 1893, Caroline Platt filed maps of the first subdivision of land into residential building lots. There were two sections to the map.

One was on the west side, near Country Lane Drive, and the other on the east side. This area is now called Field of Five, in Sunken Meadow State Park. Today, the park boasts facilities for biking, horseback riding, watersports, and general recreation. There are also three miles of beaches on Long Island Sound, as well as a three-quarter-mile boardwalk and six miles of hiking trails.

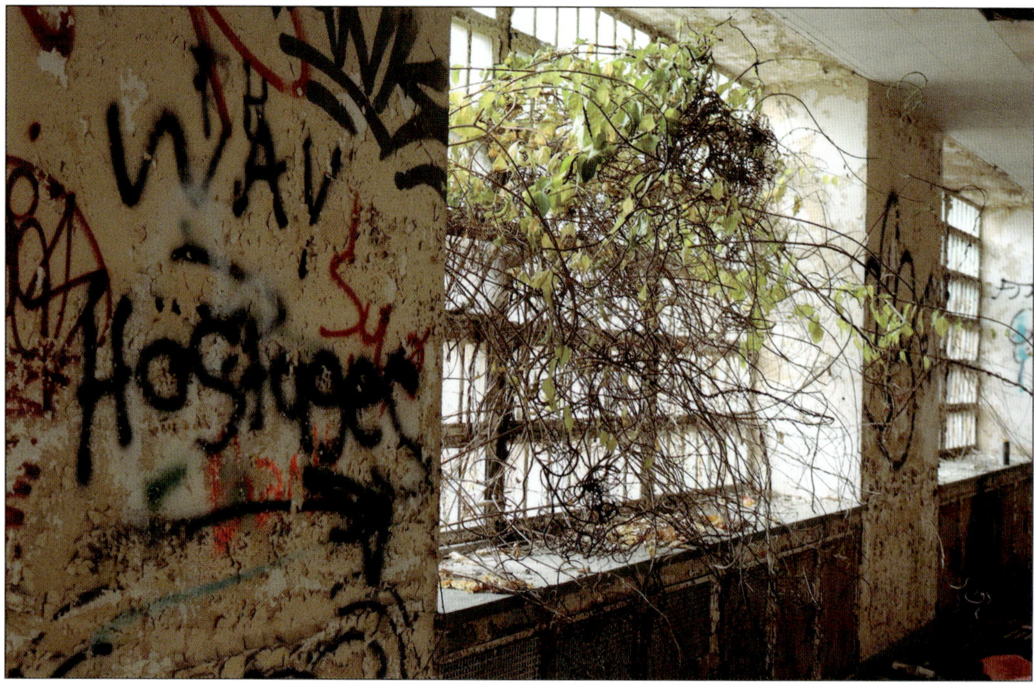

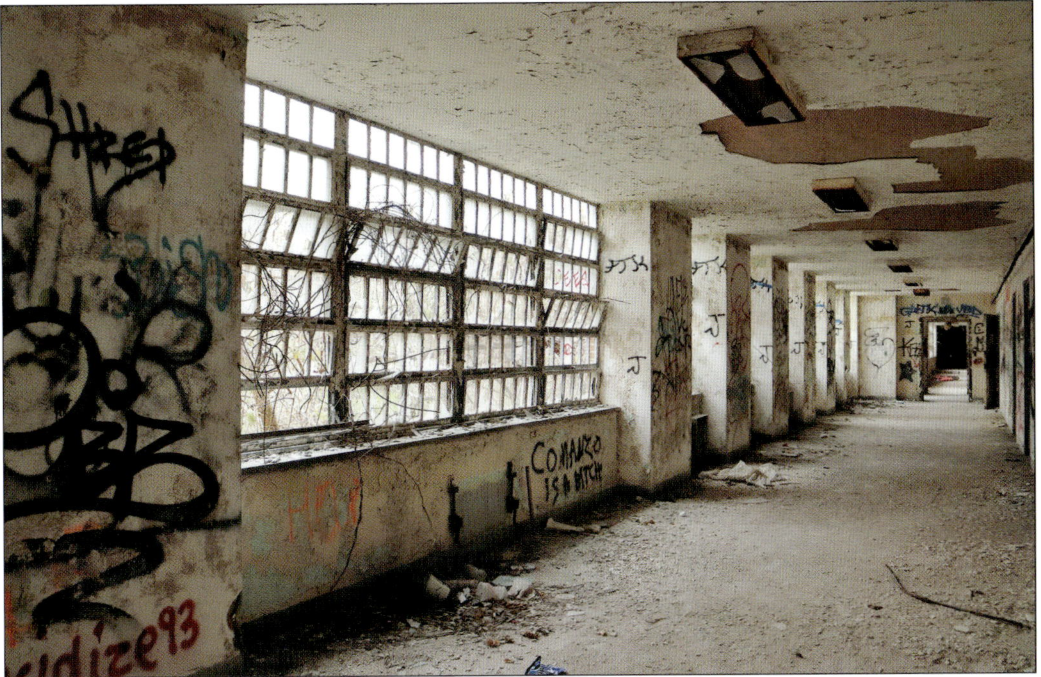

In 1896, the State of New York bought both the grounds and the buildings for $1. This was due in large part to the corruption and graft during construction of the facility, which led to outlandish spending. This is when the facility in Kings County became known as the Long Island State Hospital.

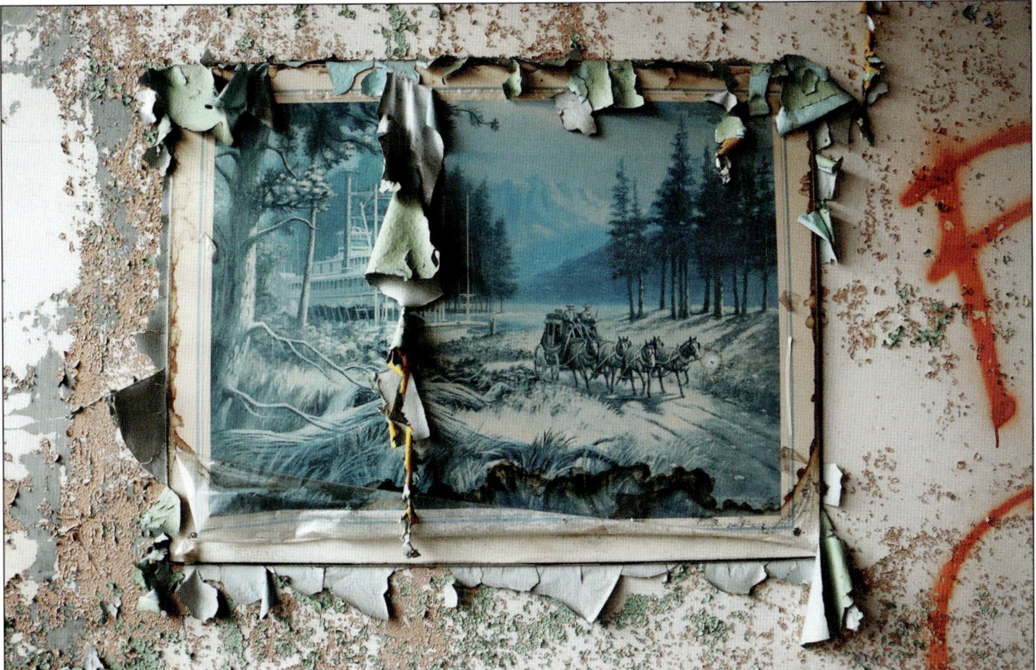

In 1896, the School of Nursing was established. On October 1 of the same year, Long Island State Hospital became a state institution when Kings County commissioners transferred the hospital in Brooklyn, together with this institution, to the state.

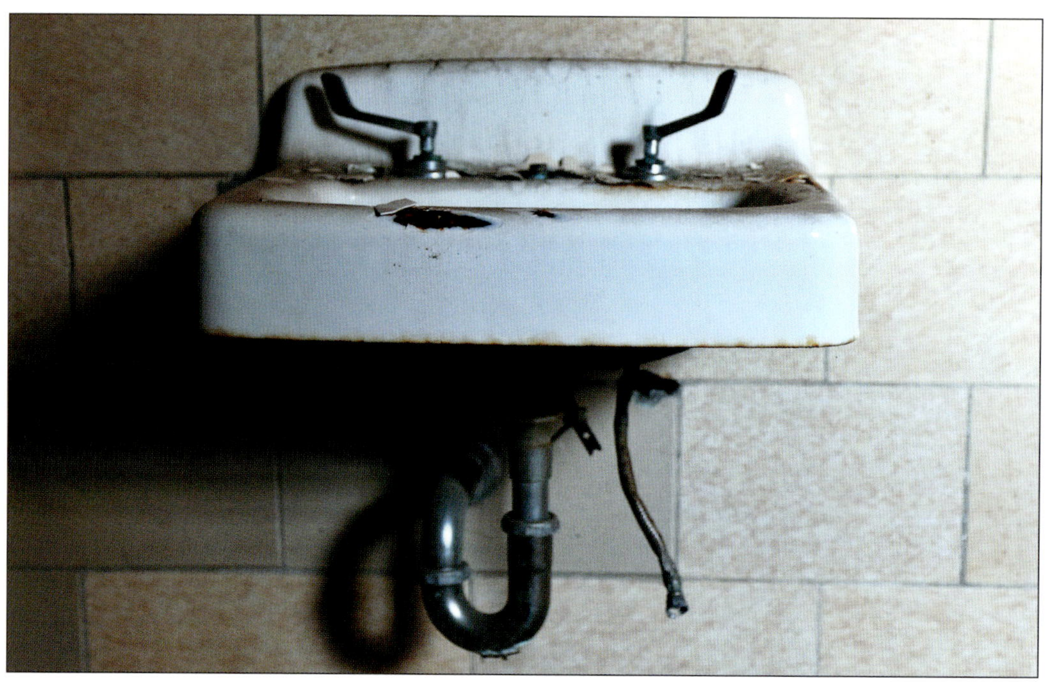

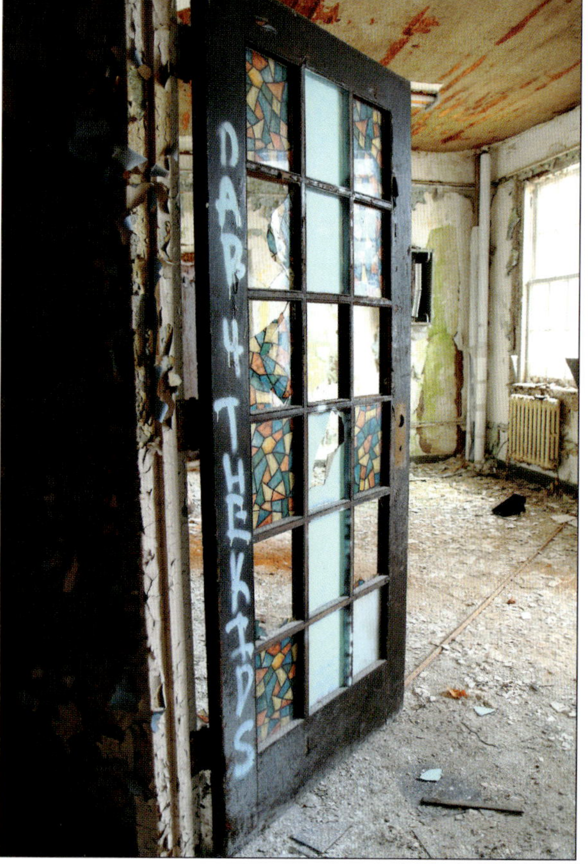

With conditions at the hospital being poor, in 1896, the state legislature appointed Hugo Hirsch as a special investigator. Through his investigation, control of the Flatbush asylum and the St. Johnland branch were also transferred to the state in October. This is said to have begun a new and hopeful area for Kings County Asylum and its branch. The following photographs were taken on Wards 60–65.

The year 1897 brought new leadership to the facility, with a new director, Oliver Dewing, who had been serving as the general superintendent. A new house for the director was built, and Dr. Dewing moved in and assumed his new role. The actual move was held up for a year until suitable accommodations could be provided.

By this time, it was becoming increasingly difficult to administer the Kings Park branch from the offices in the Flatbush hospital. The governing board of the hospital felt that the general superintendent, Dr. Oliver Dewing, should move to Kings Park since it was developing rapidly, while the Brooklyn facility was at a standstill.

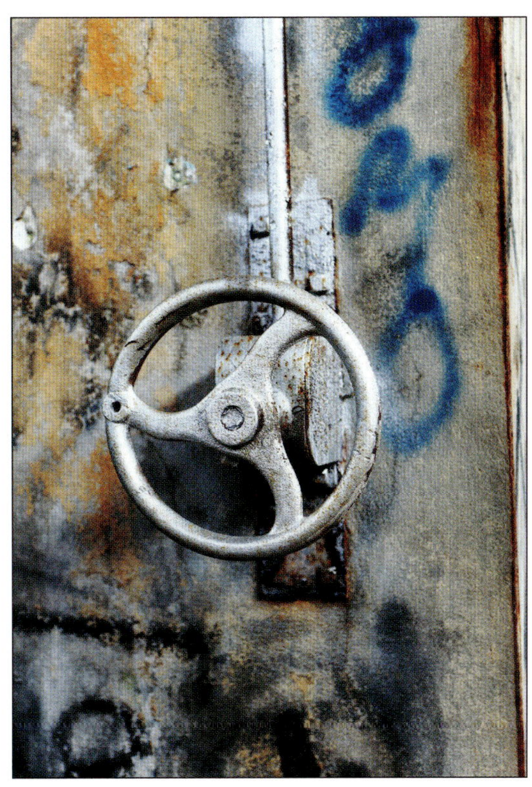

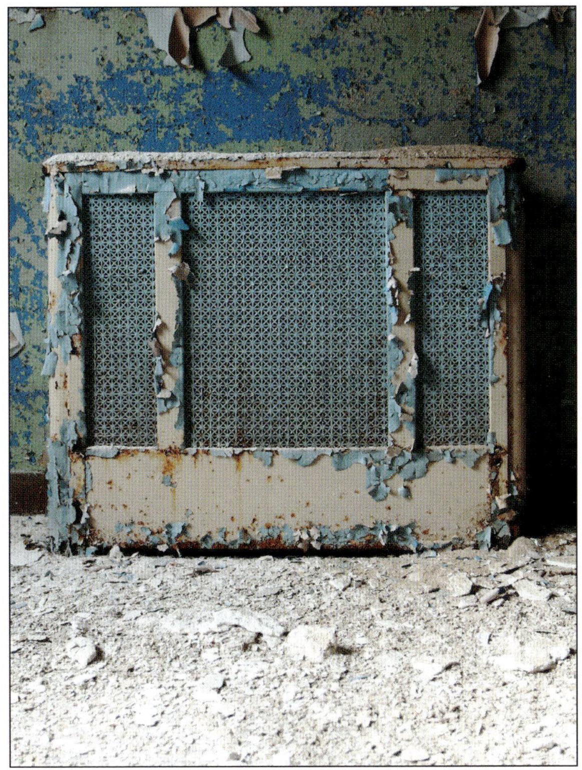

One of the first things Director Dewing began to advocate for was separate employee buildings. He felt this would attract more staff, as the facility was understaffed, as well as provide more beds for patients. The following photographs were taken on Wards 101–128, the kitchen and dining hall.

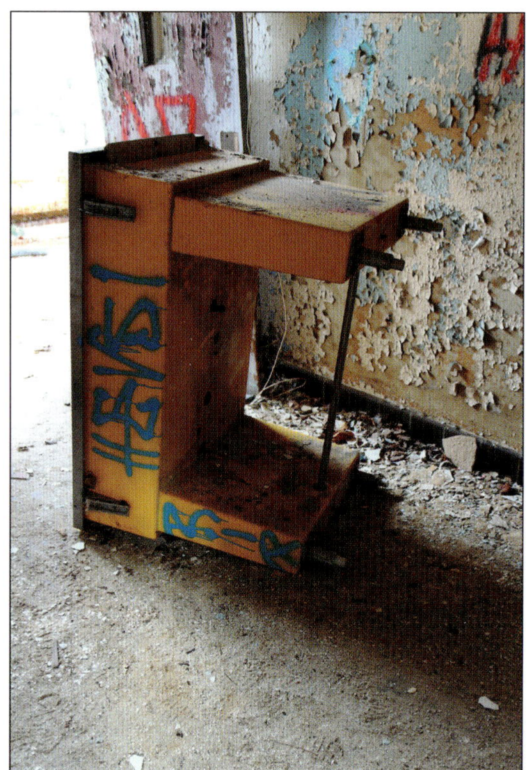

Until this time, employees lived alongside the residents and did not have anywhere but the local bars to socialize or get away from the job. In the late 1890s, a map covering the second subdivision in Kings Park was filed the county clerk's office.

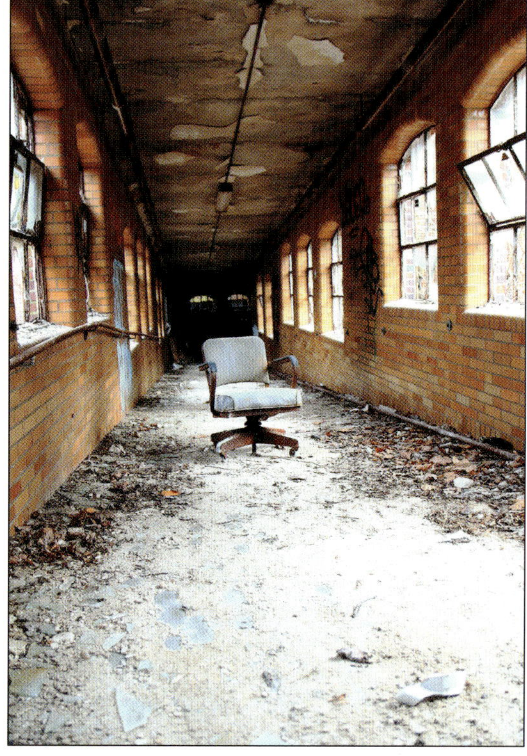

The area delineated on this map, which was in the following years refiled several times, was called "agricultural city" and covered 734 acres in the old Northport Road/Meadow Road area. By 1897, another subdivision map was filed. This map included an 11-acre triangular tract along the south side of St. John Road. Today, this area is between Birch and Hemlock Roads.

Three

Into the 1900s

It is locally well known that in the late 1940s, *Ripley's Believe it or Not!* announced that Kings Park had more bars per capita than anywhere else in the nation. Less well known was a geographical study of over 700 towns in the United States that found that Kings Park also had the most health care workers per capita. These facts were due to the presence of Kings Park State Hospital, an 873-acre campus to care for people suffering from mental illnesses.

It is difficult to imagine a built-up place more idyllic than the hospital: a large cluster of attractive buildings surrounded by open farm fields and wooded hills. The hospital had the right amounts of sweet ingredients: a shady boulevard with a grassy median; vistas of Long Island Sound; granite curbs; green, old-fashioned streetlights; and about a hundred institutional buildings that were diverse and yet in harmony with each other. Also important, the hospital lacked features such as signs, large parking lots, and overhead wires that lessen the appeal of many modern communities. Kings Park State Hospital was attractive and visually unique. This was due to the juxtaposition of three phenomena: the design of the buildings and grounds, its location on rolling terrain overlooking Long Island Sound and the Nissequogue River, and its large greenbelt of woods and farmland.

—David Flynn

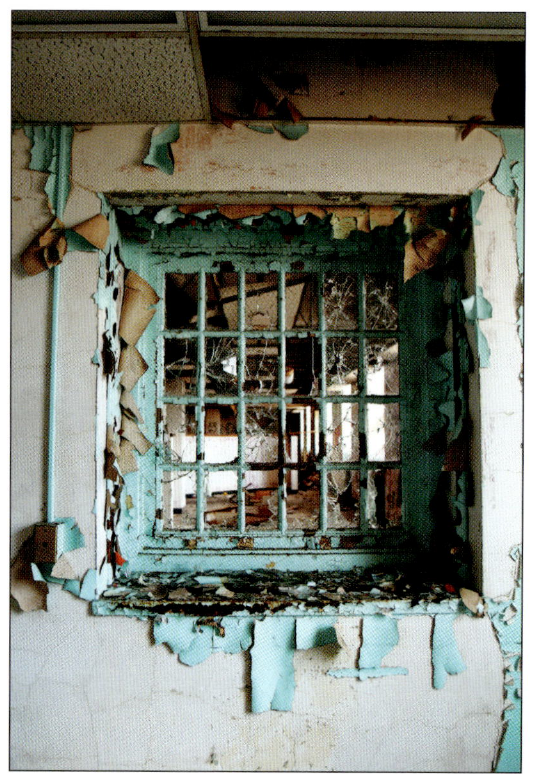

In 1898, the facility had a training school to give instruction to the employees on policy and patient care. The days were long, with ward employees working 12-hour shifts six days a week. During the day, each employee was responsible for eight patients, and at night the ratio switched to each being responsible for the care of 43. These photographs were taken on Wards 60–65.

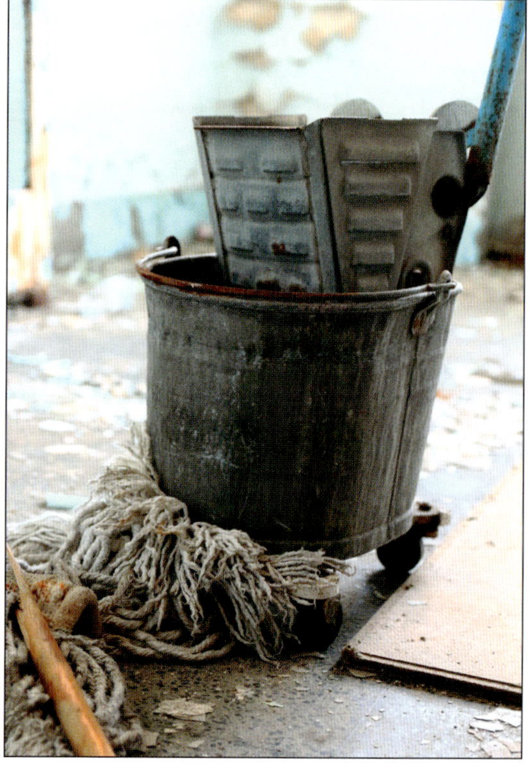

Men received $30 a month and women $25. Their job consisted of what they called "therapy." This meant keeping patients busy with work in all the trade shops and maintaining the facility.
In 1898, the fourth department was developed and was more significant than the first three. It was the first that had a number of houses built and the first to have residential streets built as well.

These cottages of various sizes, once completed, were promptly occupied by patients transferred from Flatbush. Until then, houses in the area were located on existing country roads. A real estate company known as the Kings Park Improvement Company bought about 50 acres from the Terrell family and subdivided the land into 100 lots and eight streets. The following photographs were taken on Wards 101–128, the kitchen and dining hall.

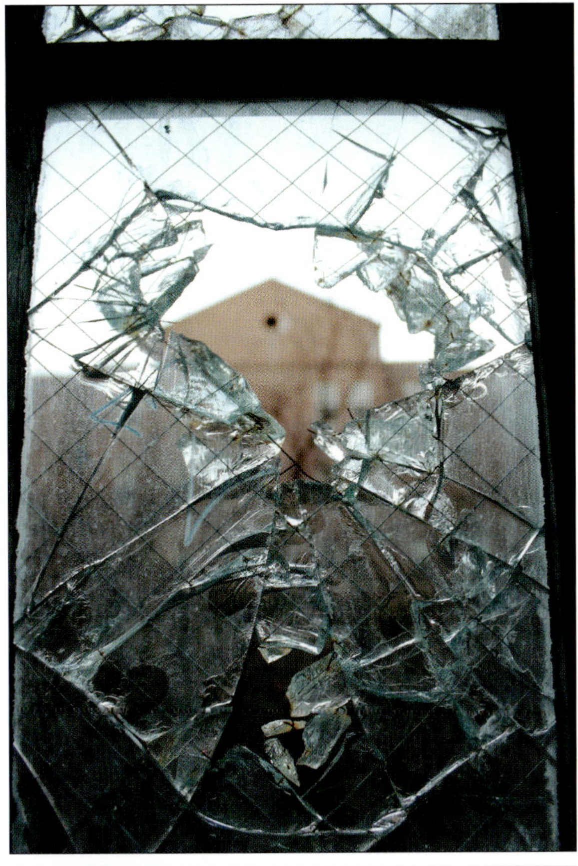

In 1896, a new and updated telephone system was installed, which connected all parts of the Kings Park facility to the general and medical offices in Flatbush. The first fire alarm system was also installed around this time; however, it was not operational by the end of the year, since the company that installed it had not furnished the needed gongs.

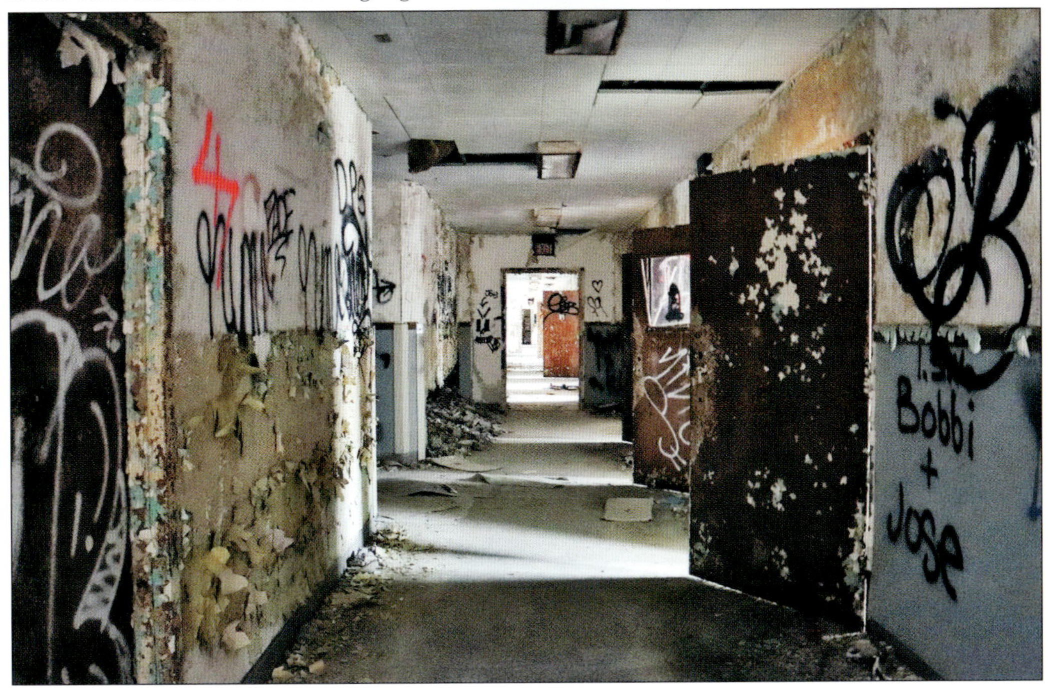

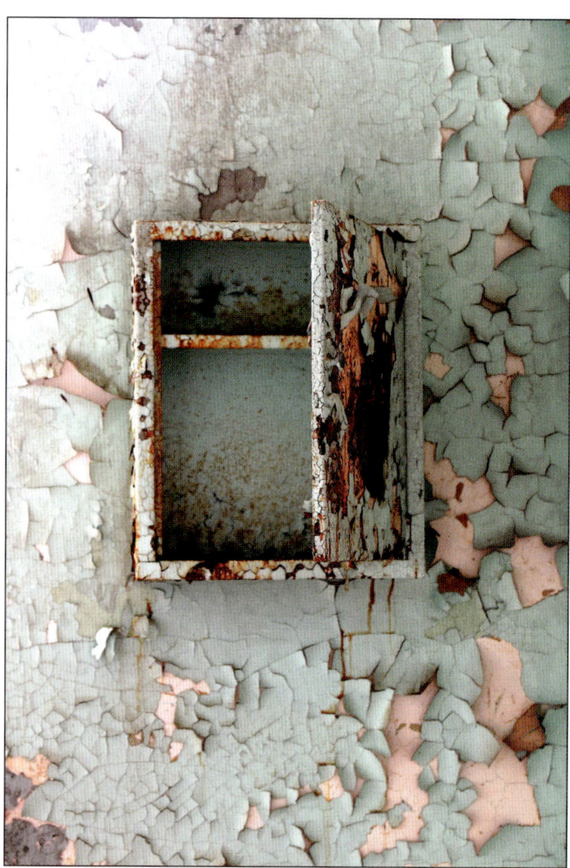

The land was located north of East Northport Road and South Main Street. By 1903, nine new homes were built along with Dawson Avenue and part of Lou Avenue. These new additions had Kings Park feeling more like a village, as opposed to just a few houses built in the same area.

The canal, which had been dug some years earlier, was improved to facilitate delivery of coal by barge to the powerhouse. Several 6,150-watt boilers were installed in the powerhouse to replace older and smaller units.

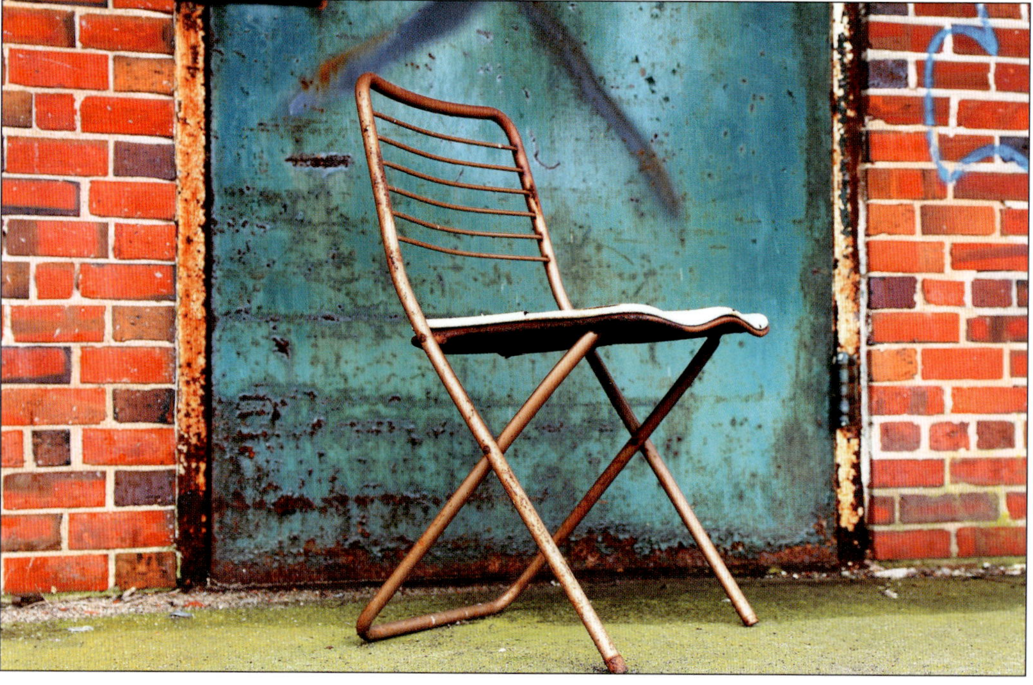

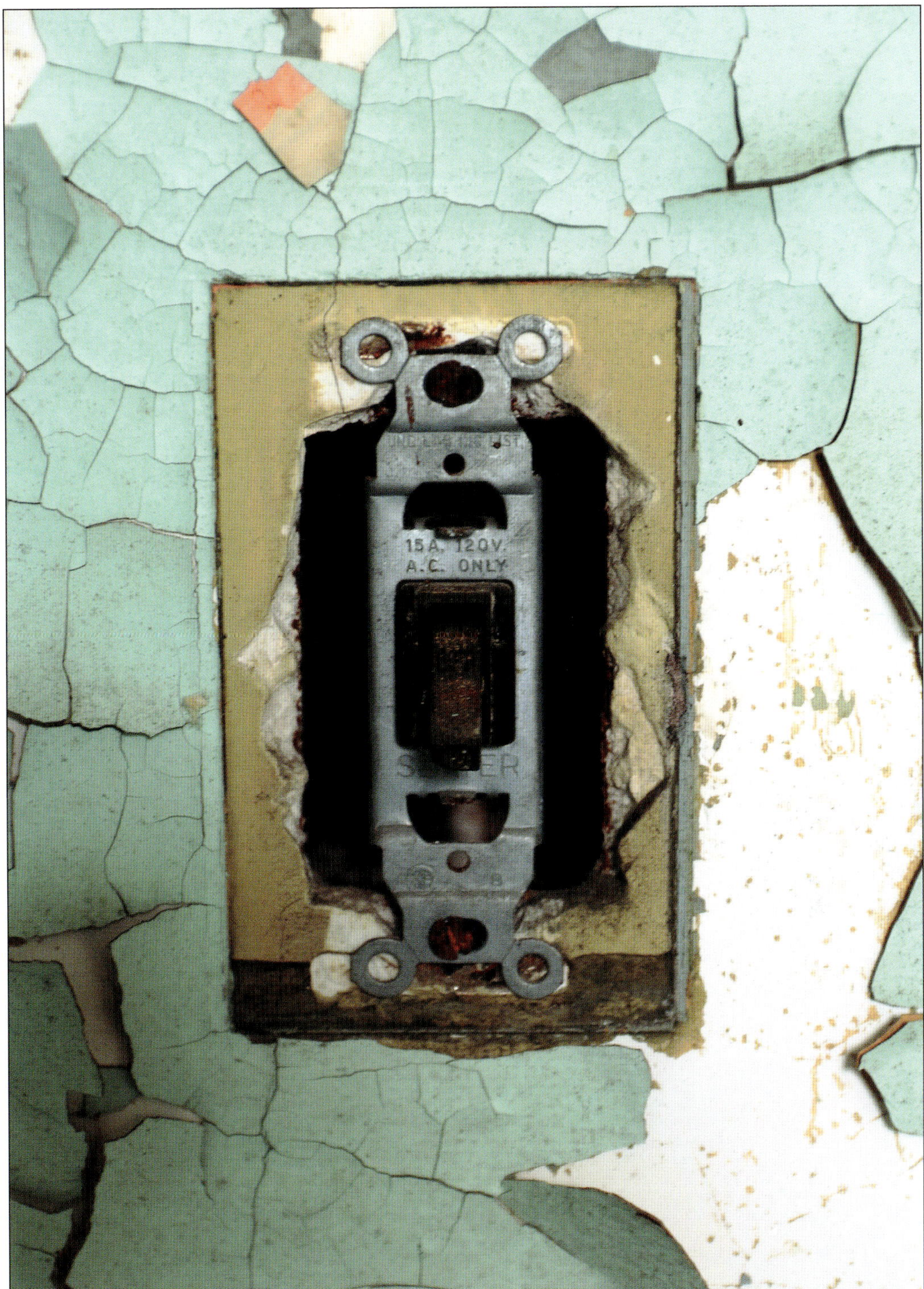

In 1897, four new buildings were completed. The construction of Buildings A, B, C, and D had begun in 1893. Also completed that year were two reservoirs, replacing the original water supply from wells near the superintendent's residence.

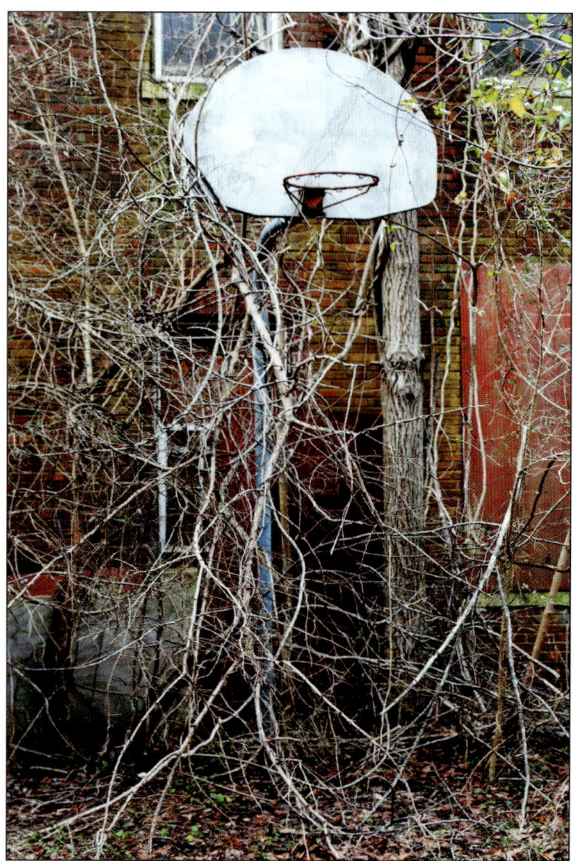

Until 1897, all patients coming to the Psych Center had been admitted in Brooklyn and transferred to Kings Park. The superintendent's report for that year states that patients were being admitted directly to the branch. The following photographs were taken on Wards 81–84.

It was even considered desirable that such patients as those received at Flatbush were removed as soon as possible to Kings Park, since a greater amount of room, better air quality, and a better environment were more conducive to speedy recoveries.

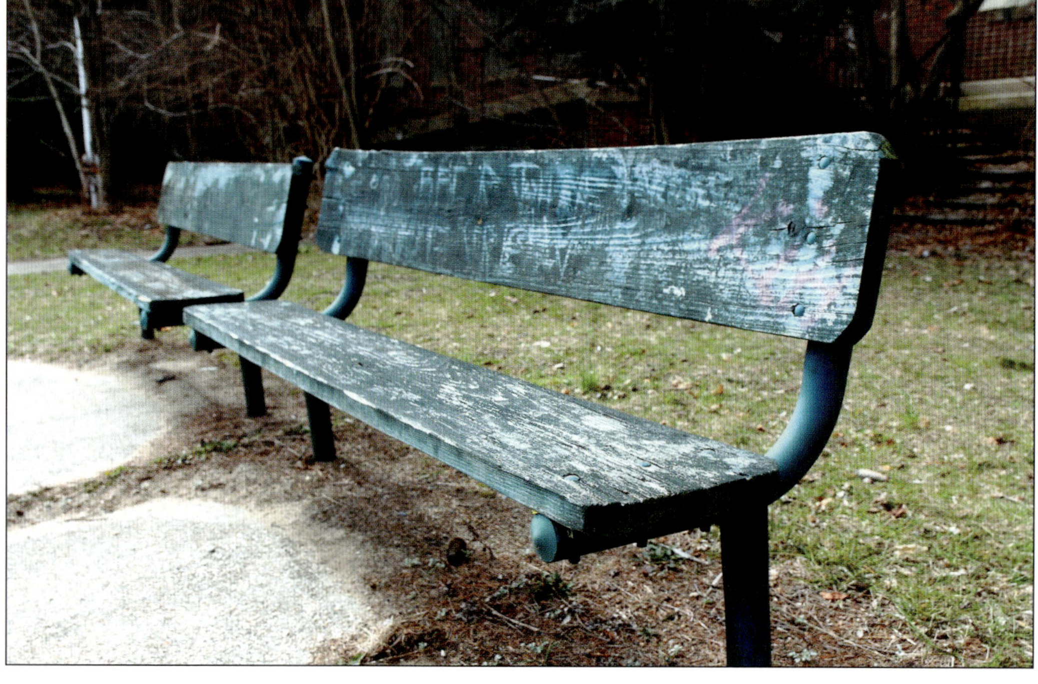

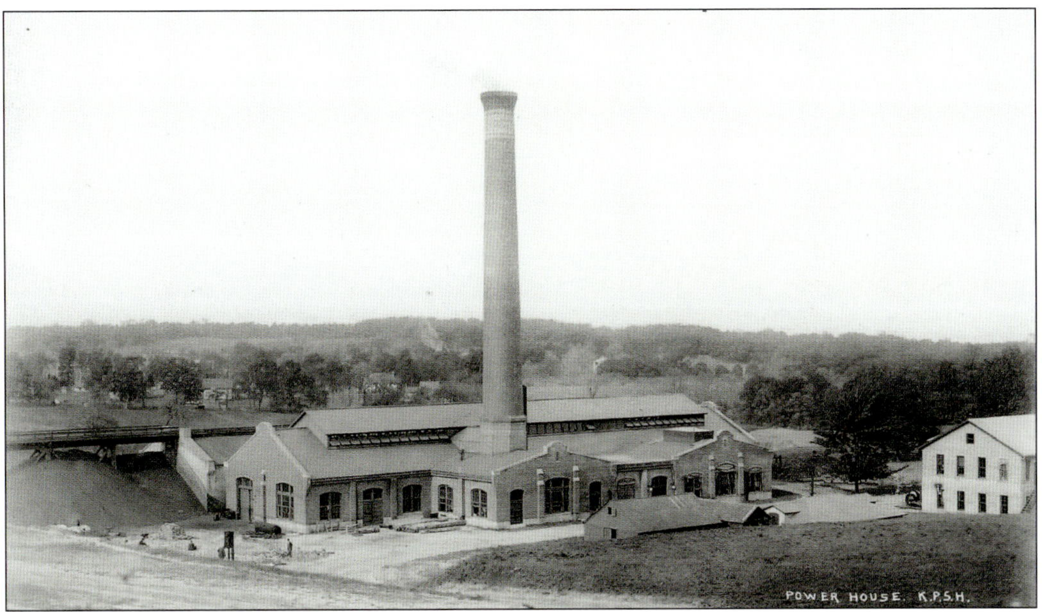

In 1897, Dr. Oliver Dewing wrote of his concern for the welfare of the employees of Kings Park Psychiatric Center, claiming there had not been any significant improvement to their social needs. He pointed out that no other hospital in the state "stands so in need of such provision since there is no city or even village nearby where employees can get away." These photographs show the powerhouse on the facility campus. (Courtesy of the Leo P. Ostebo Kings Park Heritage Museum.)

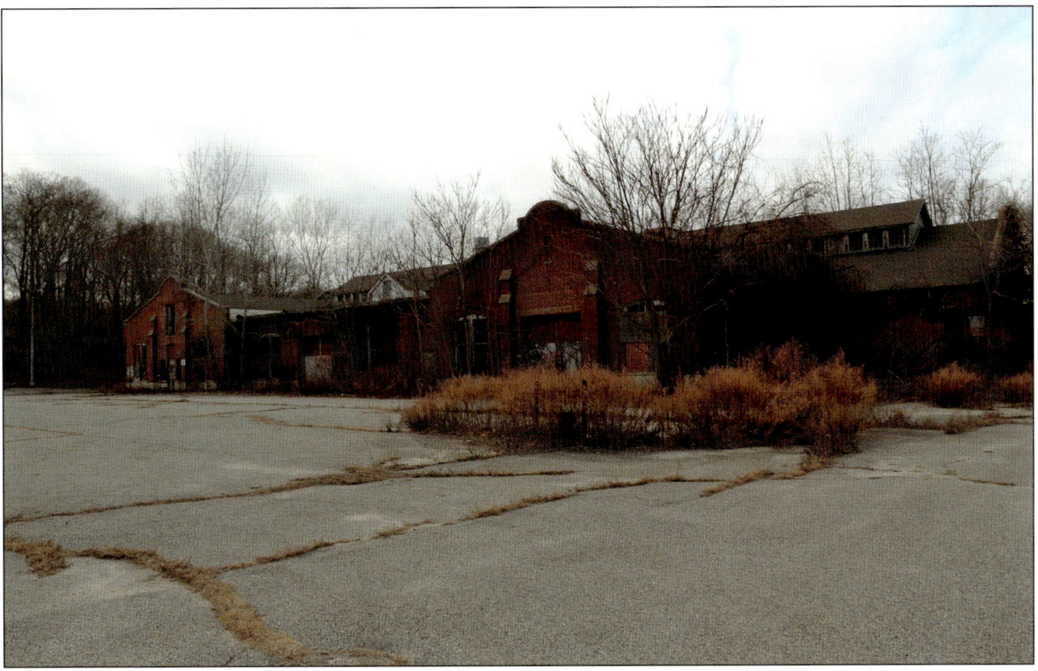

Dr. Dewing continued: "The department at Flatbush where the old buildings, defective plumbing and undesirable environment of the hospital, situated as it is in the immediate neighborhood of the penal and charitable institutions of Kings County, is certainly not such as to furnish the best surroundings for those mentally affected."

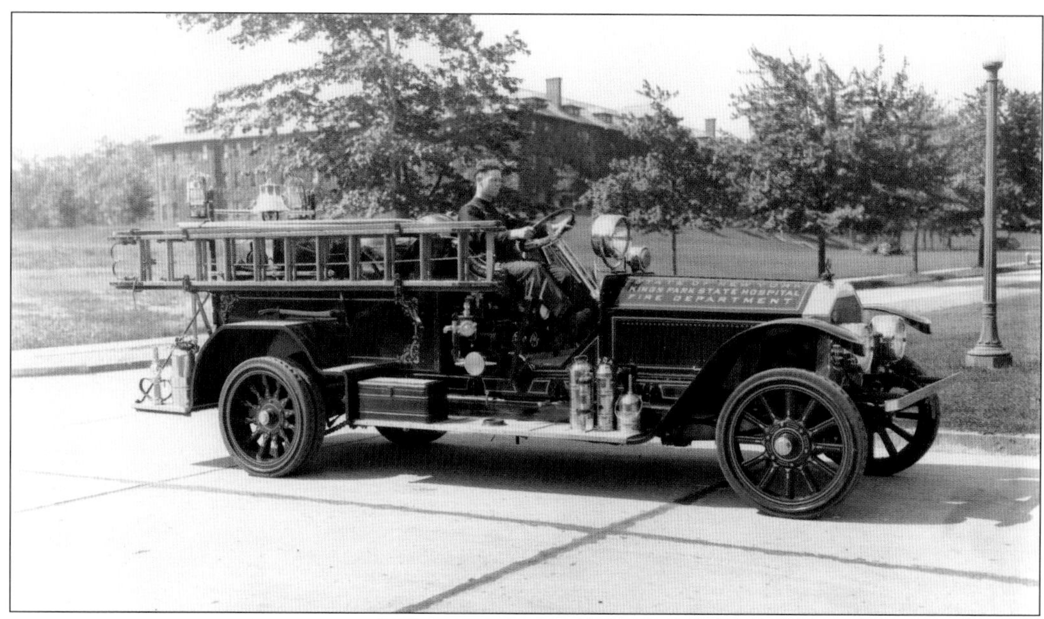

On September 30, 1897, a training school for nurses was arranged, and 17 students (all hospital employees) were admitted. The methods of teaching consisted of weekly lectures by the medical staff, based on the textbook of Dr. Wise, along with recreation, practical demonstrations, and clinical instruction on the wards. The following photographs are of the firehouse on the facility campus. (Courtesy of the Leo P. Ostebo Kings Park Heritage Museum.)

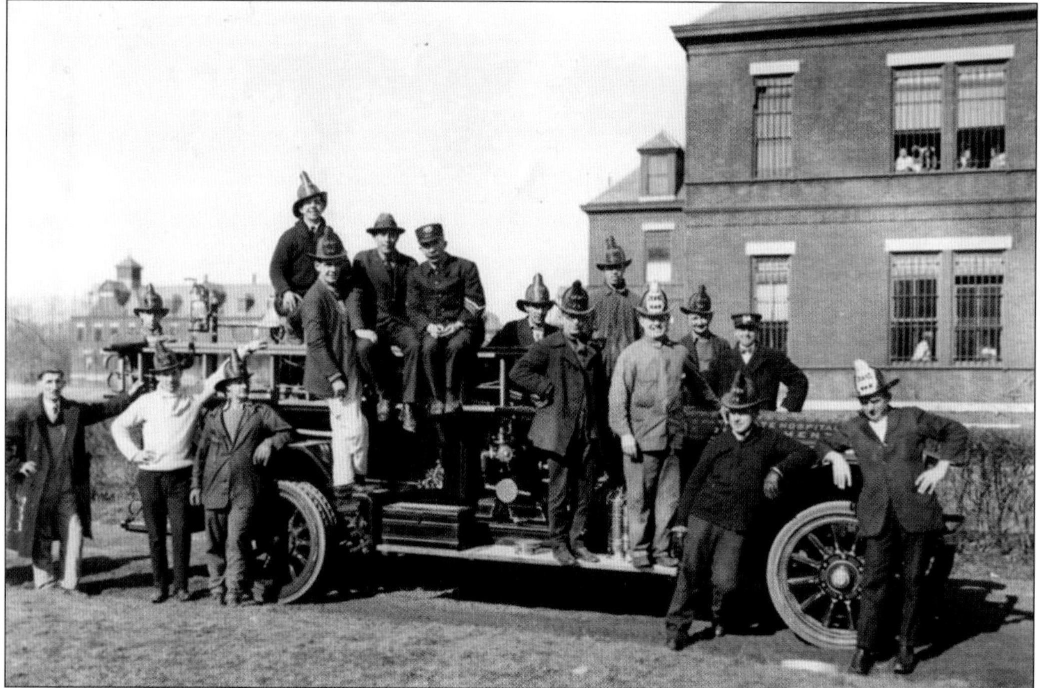

The causes of insanity at the time were classified as moral adverse conditions, such as loss of friends and business trouble, mental strain, worry at work, religious excitement, love affairs (including seduction), fright, and nervous shock. (Courtesy of the Leo P. Ostebo Kings Park Heritage Museum.)

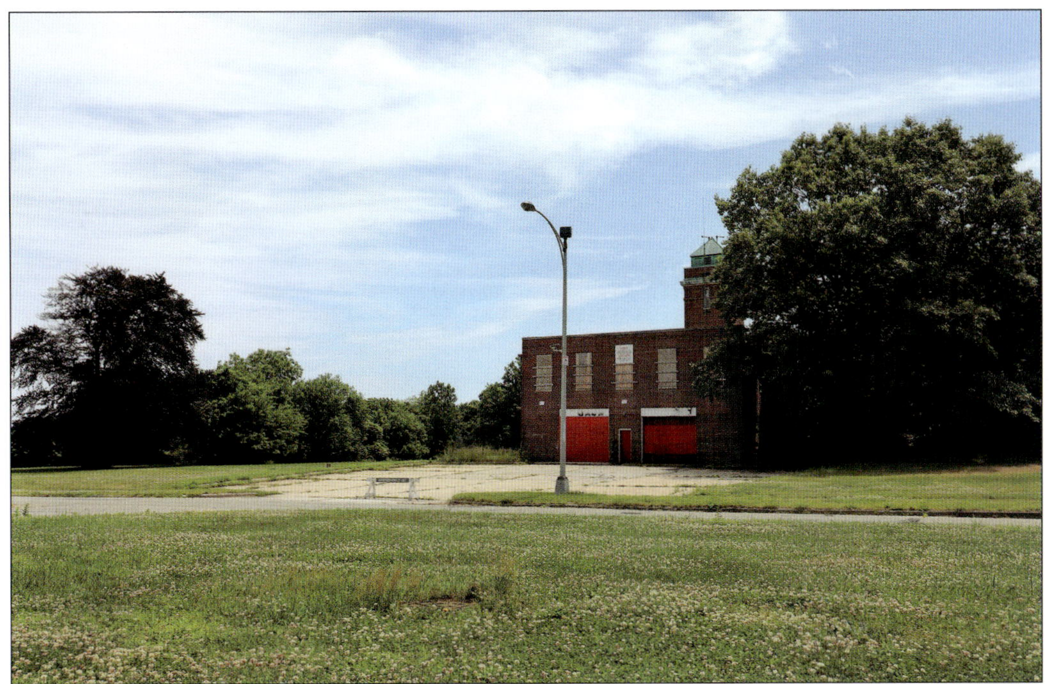

Other reasons for committal at that time included intemperance, sexual excess, masturbation, pregnancy, change of life, privation and overwork, old age, drug abuse, epidemic such as influenza, and unascertained heredity.

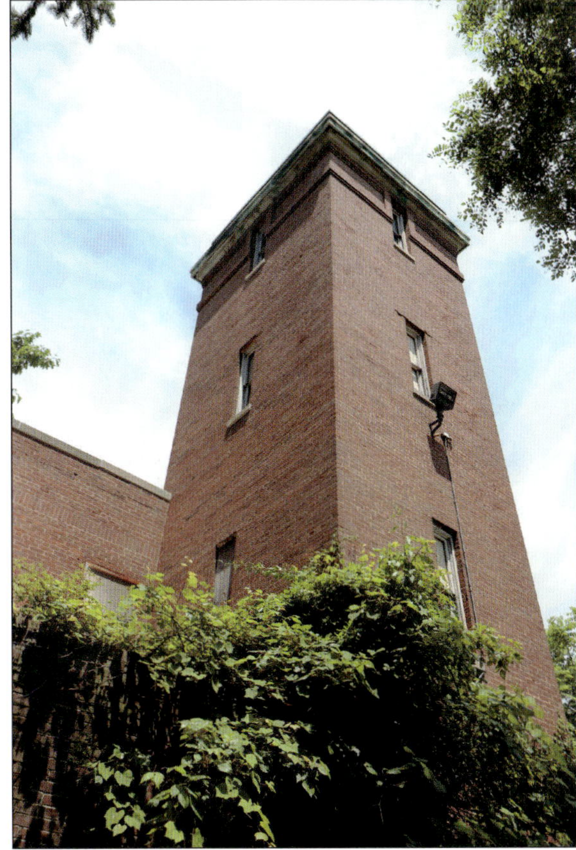

There had been 688 admissions, mostly from Kings County. Of those, 314 were native-born Americans, with 136 coming from Ireland, 112 from Germany, and the remaining coming from over 40 different countries.

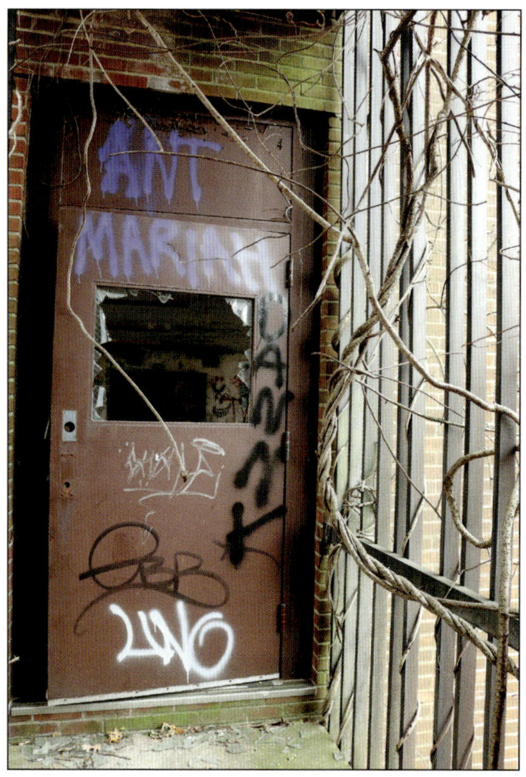

By the early 1900s, the hospital's population had grown to 2,697 patients and 454 staff members. This was greater than the entire population of the neighboring town of Smithtown. Sitting on 800 acres, the Psych Center had become a self-sufficient farming operation, complete with its own railroad spurs for the delivery of coal and supplies. This photograph was taken at the Medical/Surgery/X-Ray/Laboratory Building.

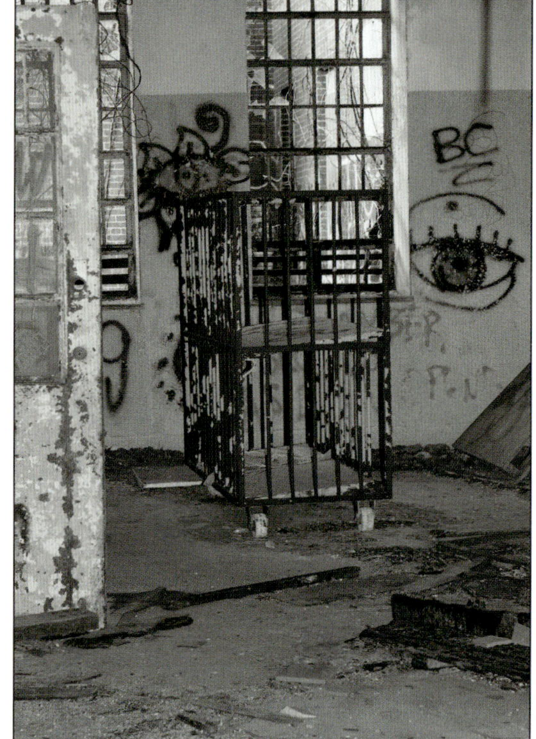

On May 1, 1900, the State of New York declared that the Long Island State Hospital at Kings Park was to be considered a facility completely separated from Flatbush. This photograph was taken on Wards 17–38.

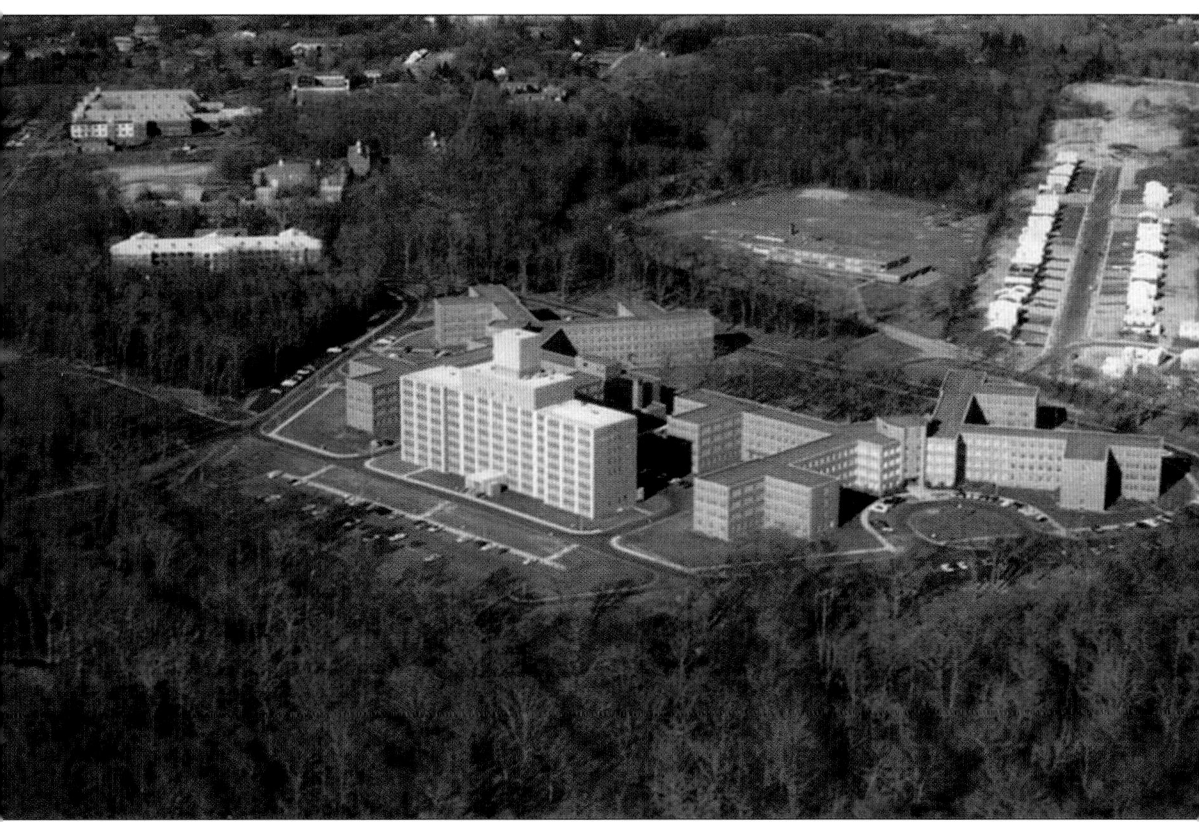

The facility was separated from the Long Island State Hospital in Kings County and became the Long Island State Hospital at Kings Park. The buildings were badly overcrowded, and the facility began the assignment of women to work on men's wards. This photograph was taken at the Medical/Surgery/X-Ray/Laboratory Building. (Courtesy of the Leo P. Ostebo Kings Park Heritage Museum.)

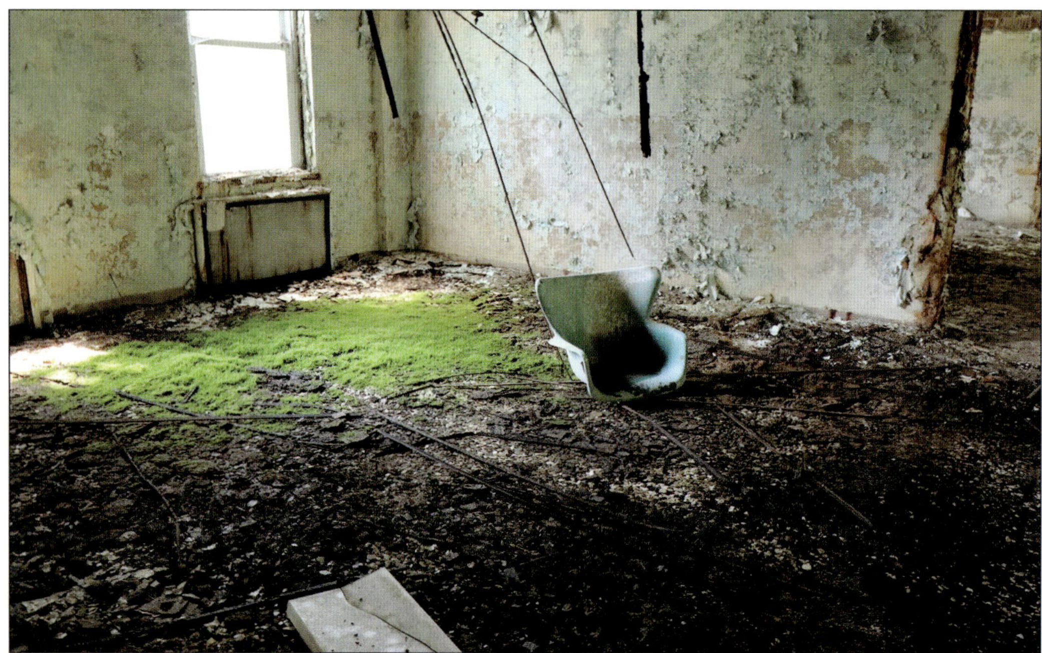

As it turned out, this seemed to work well, and it had even been reported that this led to less violence and profanity, and that the environment was more homelike and cheerful. At this time, the hospital was in the process of converting to electric power. This photograph was taken on the Mental Retardation Unit.

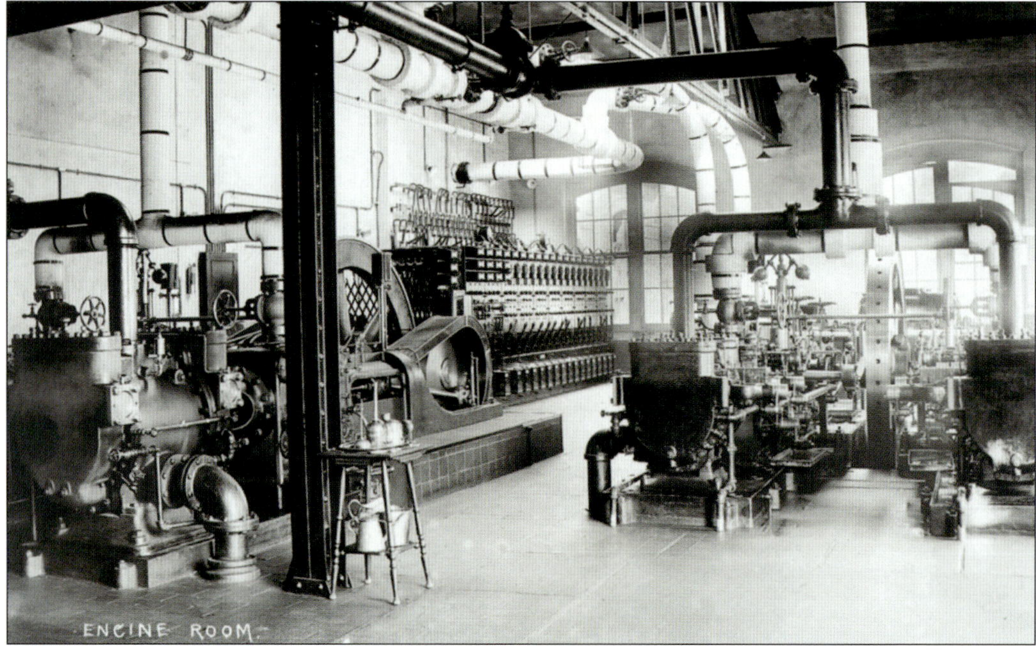

In 1901, shortly after the fire, the facility submitted a request for $800 to buy electric flat irons for the laundry and tailor shop. This was approved and added to the budget. Then, in 1903, the tailor shop sewing machines were converted to electricity. This photograph shows the engine room on the facility campus. (Courtesy of the Leo P. Ostebo Kings Park Heritage Museum.)

Four

1900–1927

The design had a pleasant combination of unity and diversity. Unity was created by the use of red brick in nearly all of the buildings. This created a sense of order and repetition, and it distinguished the hospital from the adjacent town that was built mostly of wooden homes. Diversity and interest were created by differences in the details. Buildings were added over the course of 80 years and were designed in a few distinctly different styles such as Gothic Revival, Spanish Colonial Revival, and Federal Revival. Additionally, the sizes, shapes, and setbacks of the buildings varied widely. The hospital buildings were concentrated in the middle of a large campus. The perimeter consisted of hundreds of acres of farmland and woods. This visually separated the core of the hospital from the adjacent community. It also created a strong sense of transition and anticipation when traveling from the edges to the built-up center. In addition to the noble mission of the hospital, it was a visually wonderful place that few people were fortunate enough to see.

—David Flynn

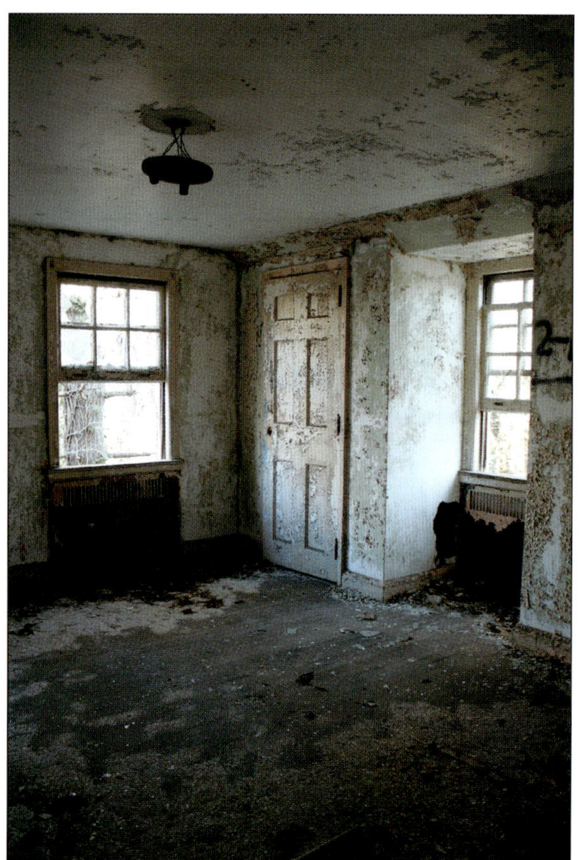

At this time, most patients were admitted to Kings County and transferred to Kings Park by train. The Long Island Rail Road maintained two passenger coaches with special locked compartments for this purpose. Beginning around 1900, Kings Park was allowed to admit patients directly rather than having all patients admitted in Brooklyn and transferred. The following photographs show the doctors' houses.

A self-sufficient farm community was established, providing work for thousands of staff members and nurses. In addition, an average of 70 percent of the patients worked various jobs on the hospital grounds.

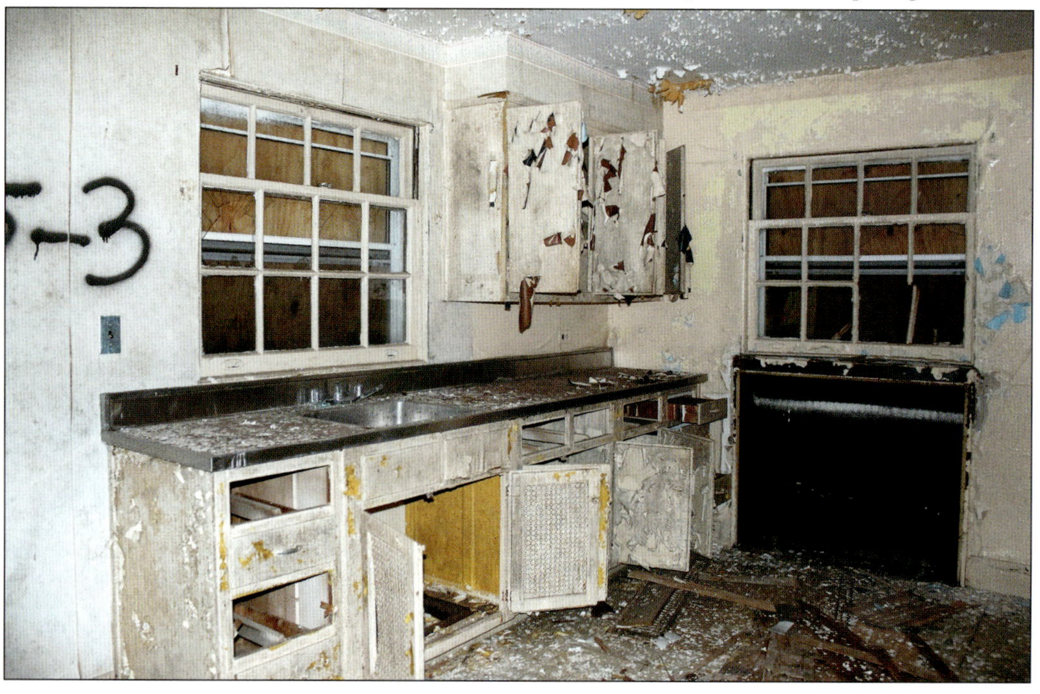

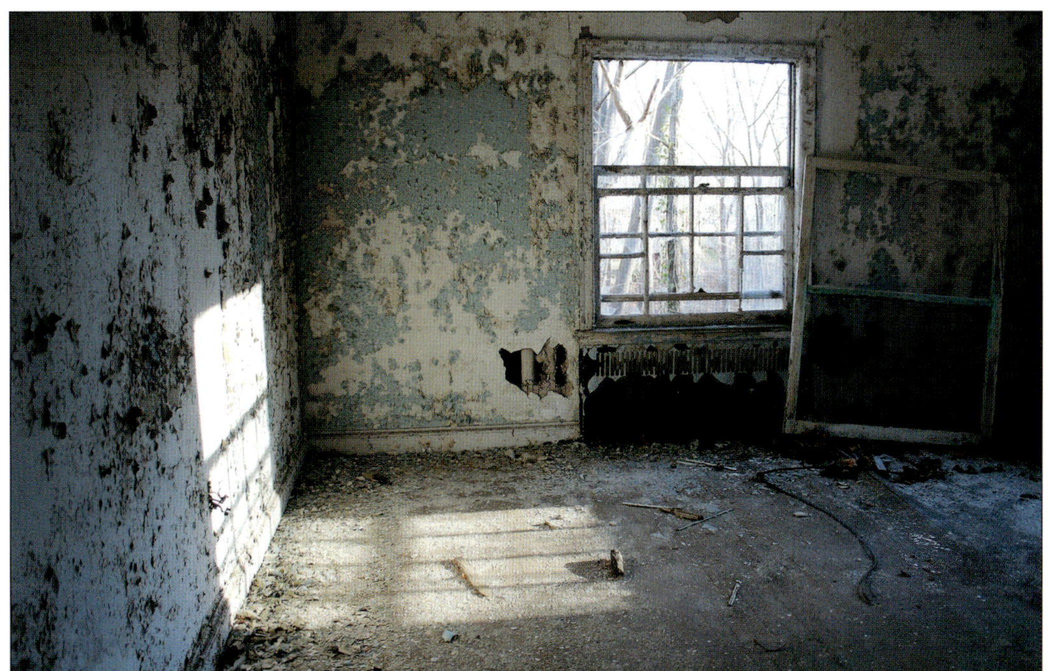

There were over 150 permanent buildings, including a laundry, bakery, library, nursing school, recreation hall, bandstand, and many repair and construction shops. Kings Park constructed its own railroad spurs in order to bring in coal and supplies from the Long Island Rail Road line.

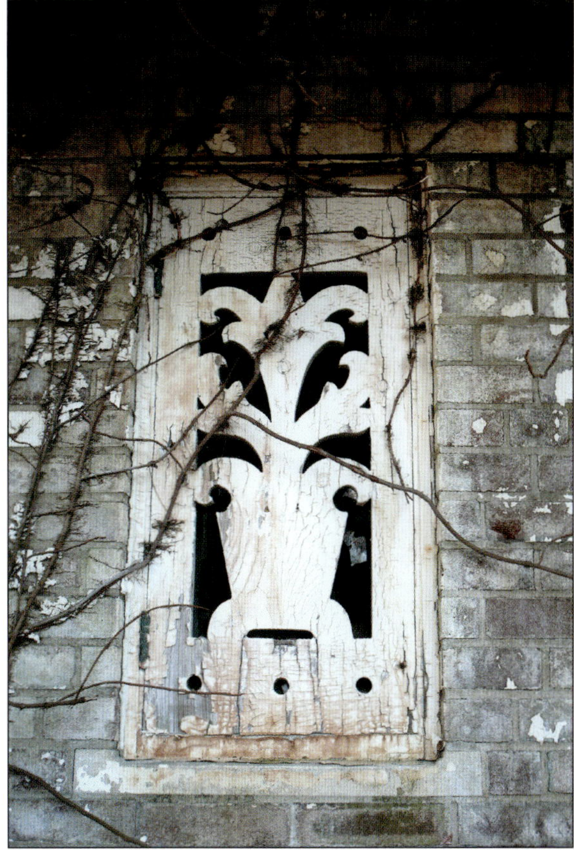

The nursing school graduation on June 20, 1903, included a demonstration of practical skills including bed making, packs, dressings, massage, and preparing and serving meals. The exercises were open to the public, which was a novelty. This tradition remained for several years, as it became popular with the locals.

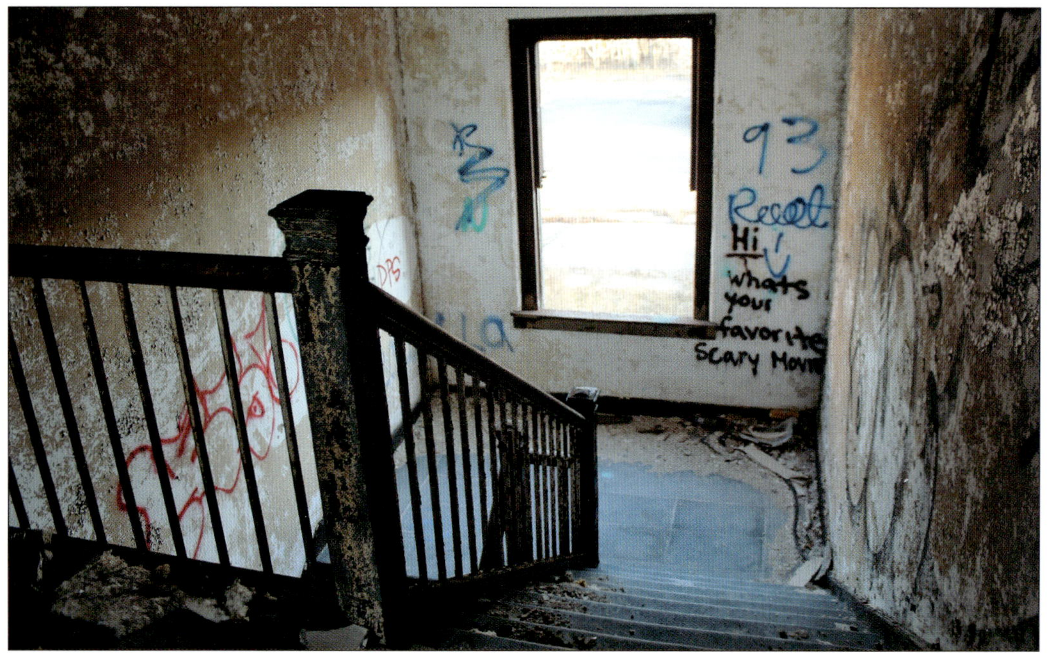

Dr. William Austin Macy became the new superintendent on June 1, 1904 , after being transferred from Willard State Hospital. He remained until his death on May 22, 1918. In 1905, the name of the facility was changed to Kings Park State Hospital. The nursing school registered with the New York Department of Education.

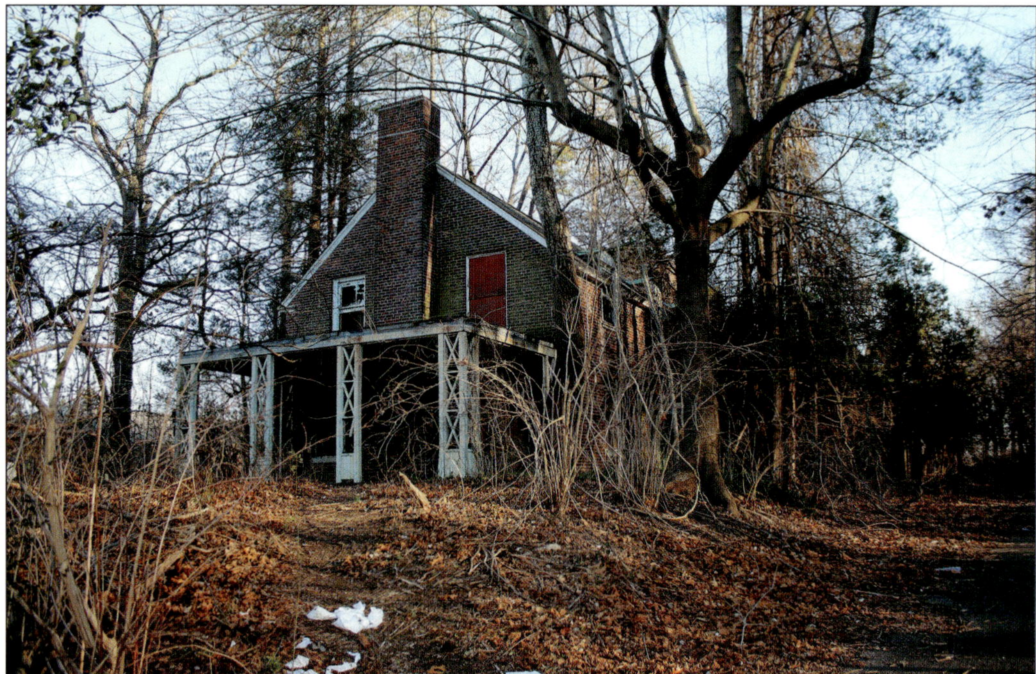

No admissions were accepted at Kings Park in 1905. In fact, 241 patients were transferred to Rochester, which had a new building. This brought the population to 2,571, which was still well over the capacity of the facility.

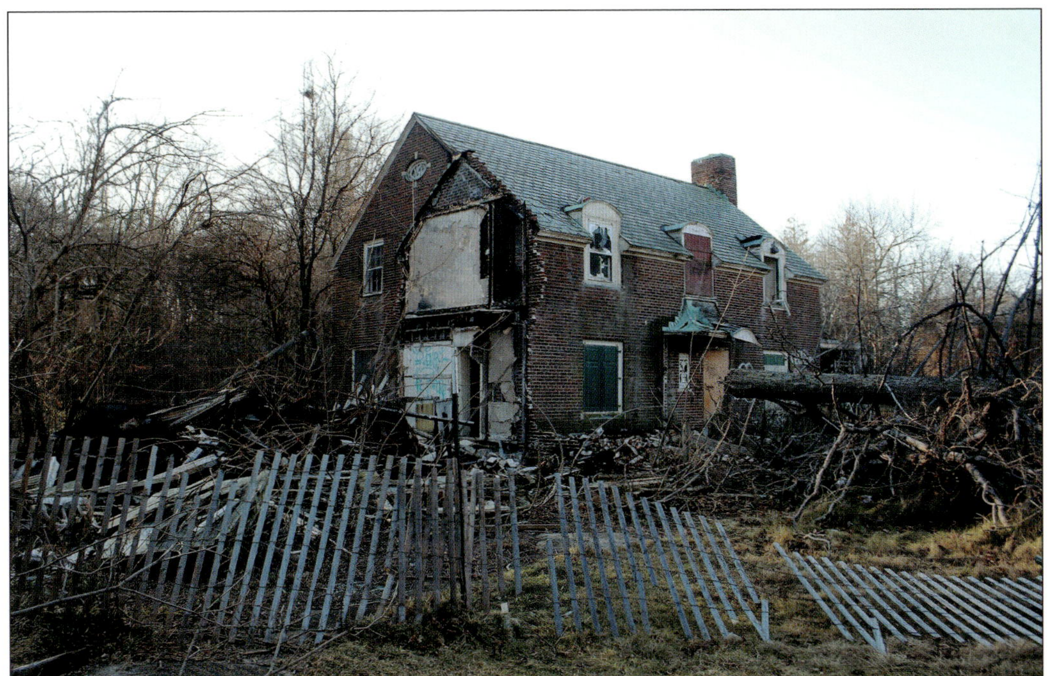

In November 1906, the laundry burned to the ground. Sparks from a switch engine ignited the fire, and with flames fanned by high winds, the building was completely destroyed along with all laundry equipment and a large amount of clothing and bed linen. Loss was estimated at $86,677.25.

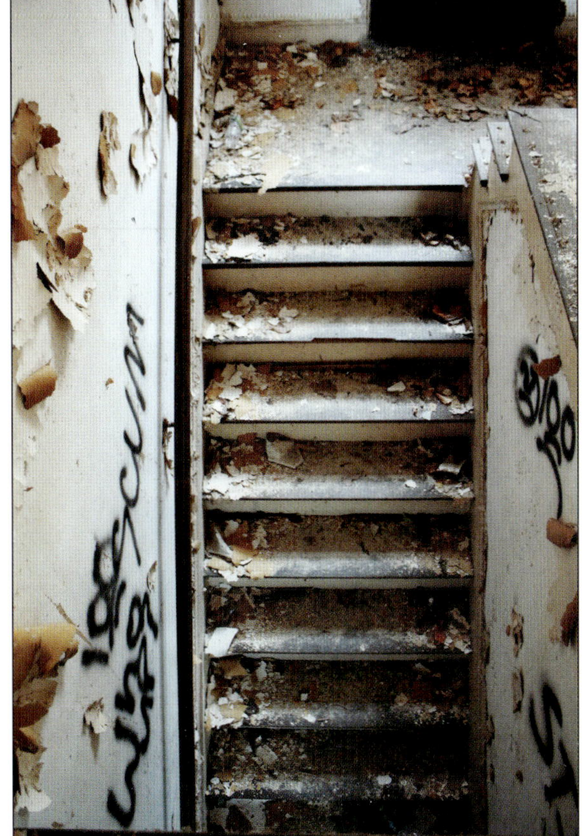

The facility's first gasoline-powered fire truck was innovative, but came with limitations. A memo had been sent to all employees asking them to not hitch rides up the boulevard since the truck could not make the grade with too many people.

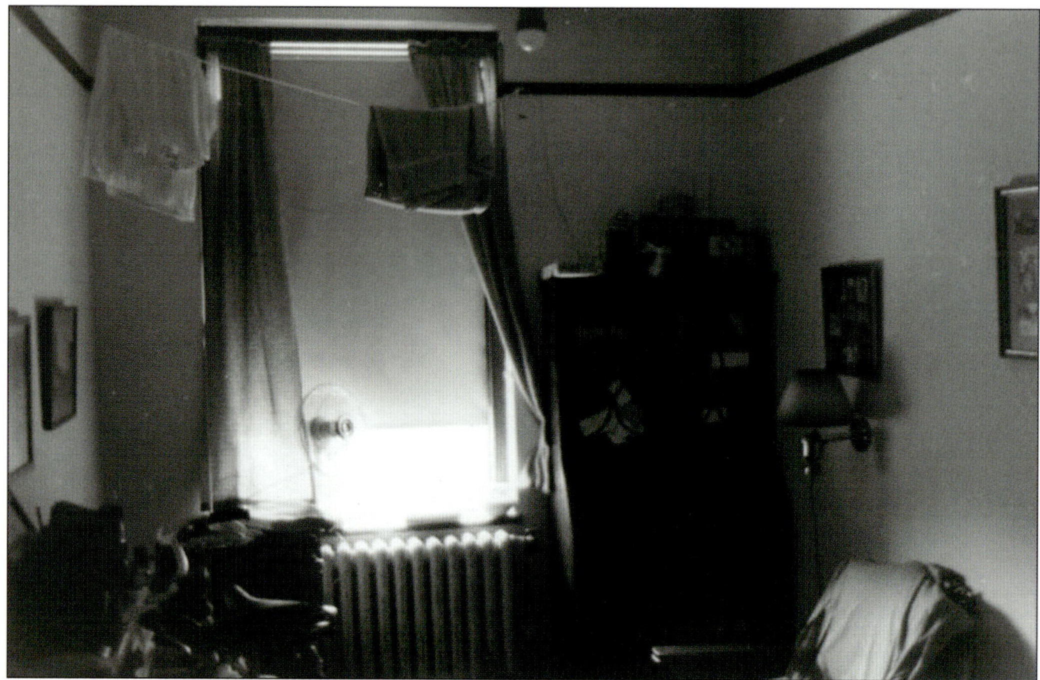

In 1907, arrangements were made for nursing students to affiliate at Bellevue so they could qualify for registration as graduate nurses. Prior to this time, the school graduates could only work as nurses in state facilities.

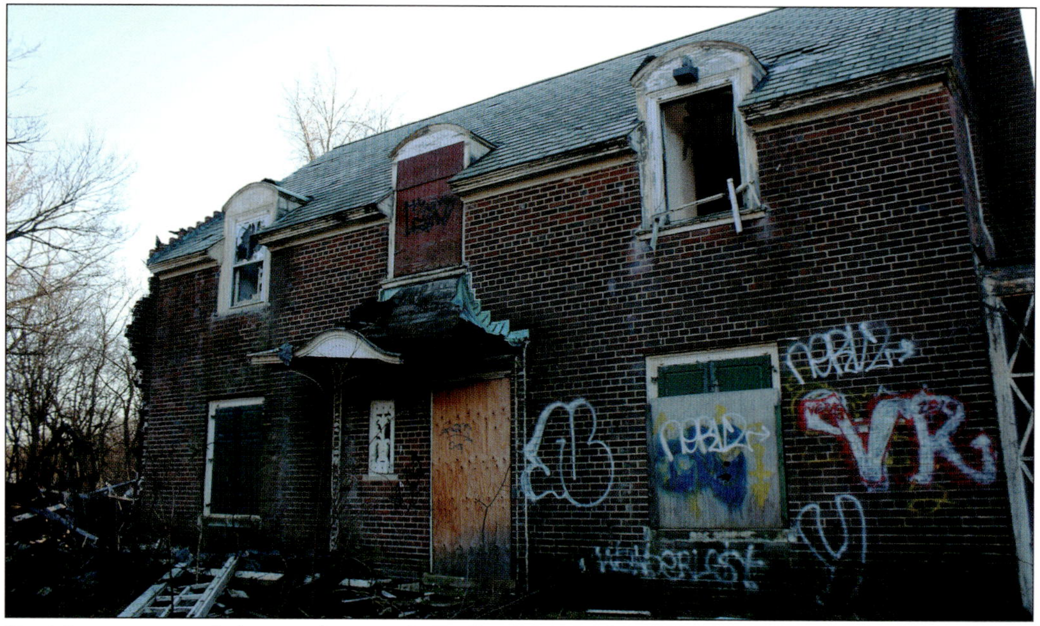

Dr. Macy requested the employee salaries be increased to be comparable to salaries in local industries. He had advertised from Canada to South Carolina and west to Indiana without any success. Although an economic depression in 1908 allowed Dr. Macy to fill staff with well-qualified people, he continued asking for improved pay scales, a pension plan, and other benefits, especially for medical personnel.

By 1910, the population had grown to 3,291, and Dr. Macy requested an expansion of the facilities. It was suggested that he transfer some of the patients to upstate facilities, but he argued that would not be therapeutic, as it would uproot patients, taking them away from visiting relatives.

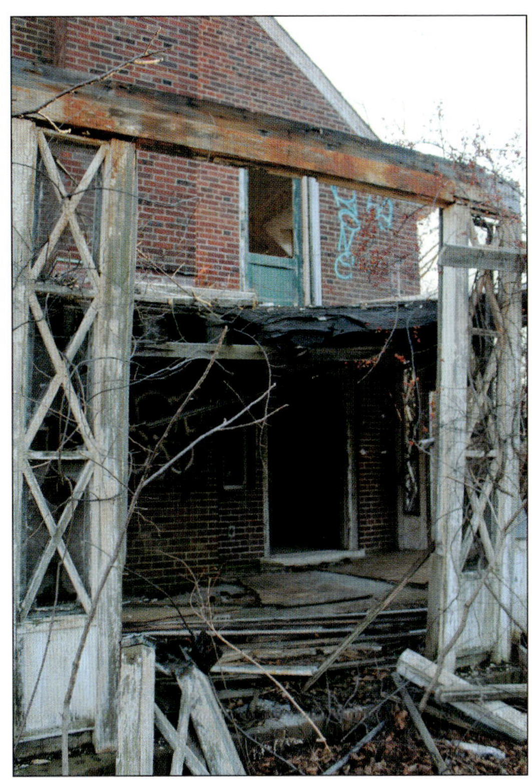

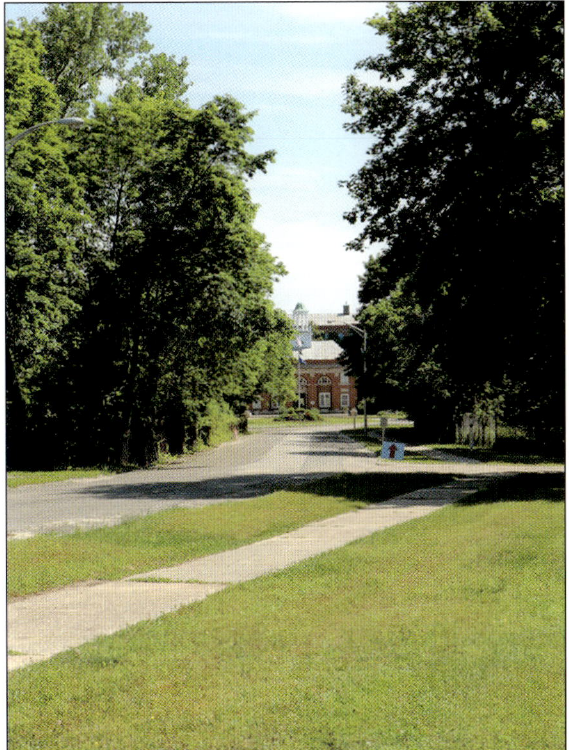

A new boiler house and laundry opened in 1910, and the following year, the nursing school appointed its first principal, Ida M. Marker, RN. The hospital continued improvements, and by 1912 purchased a moving picture machine, and then an auxetophone was purchased from the Victor Talking Machine Company to amplify sounds and supply music for dances and other entertainments.

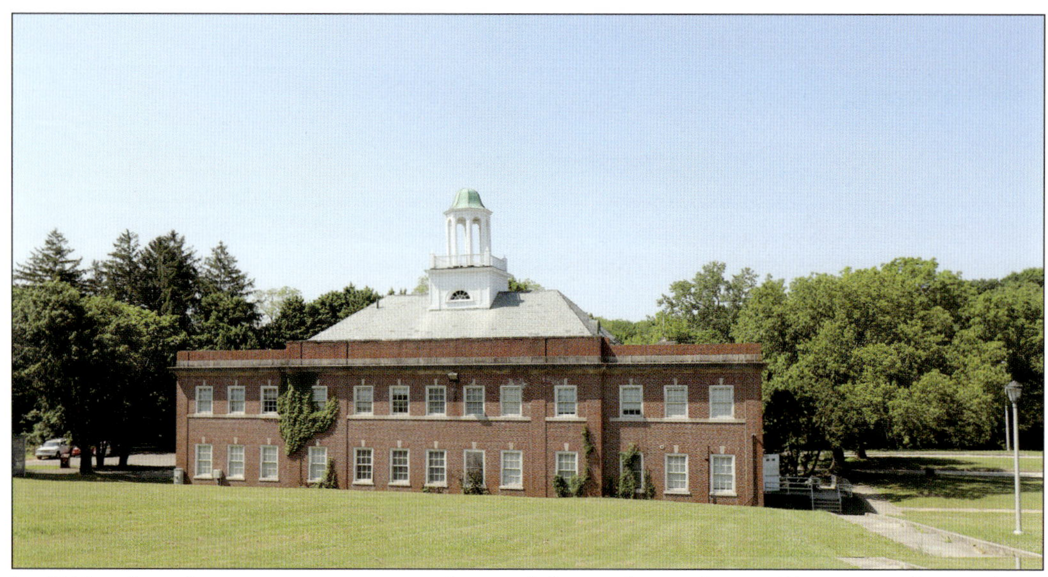

In 1913, a formal training program was designed for ward attendants. Classes met for one hour twice a week for lectures, demonstrations, and testing. All new employees were required to attend. By this time, the patient population had grown slightly to 4,000, just above capacity. Also in 1913, group tuberculosis "camps" (cottages) opened, the Kings Park Fire Company was formed, and the state opened a piggery. This photograph is of the Administration Building.

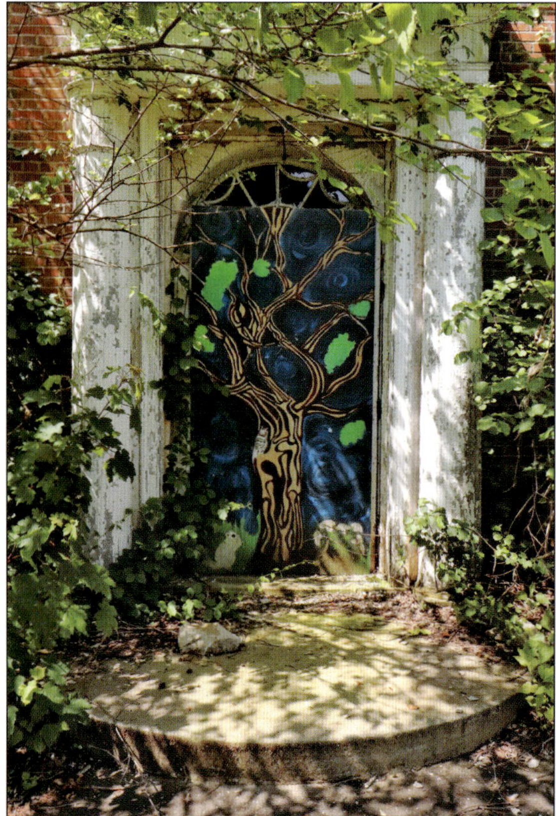

In 1916, building construction continued; however, the staff was depleted due to the Great War. The year 1917 saw the rise of outpatient services and mental hygiene clinics for teens and discharged patients in both Kings and Nassau Counties. The following photographs show the offices and patient residences.

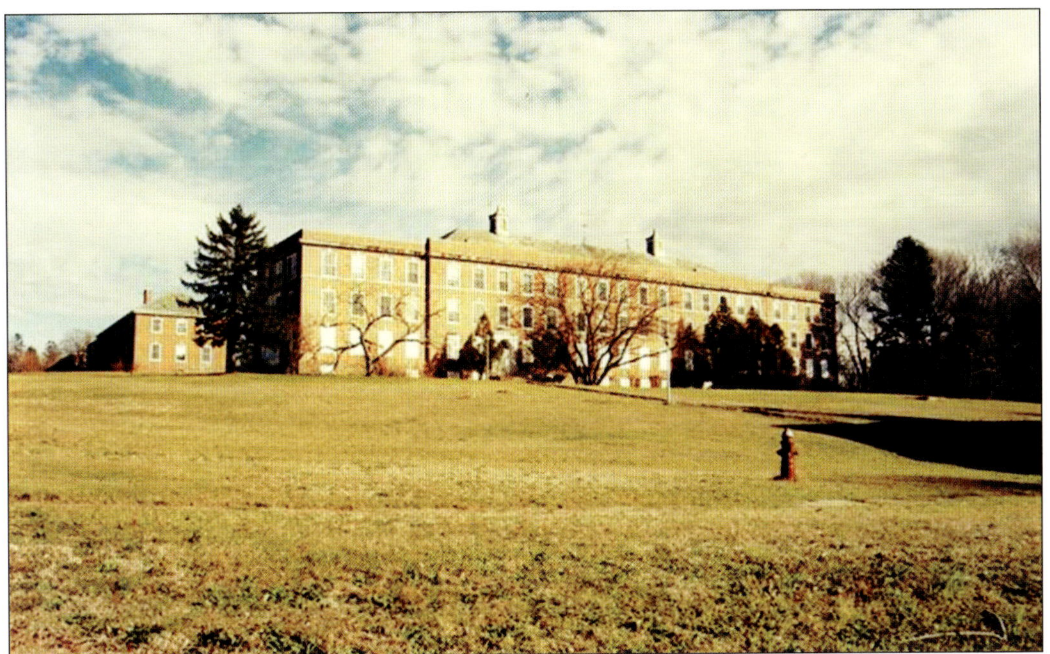

Dr. Macy, who led through the era of rapid growth, died in 1918. That same year, Macy House opened. The Spanish influenza pandemic started in September 1918 and lasted until April 1919. Often, the flu would lead to pneumonia; 537 patients and 151 employees took ill, with 58 patients and four employees dying as a result. (Courtesy of the Leo P. Ostebo Kings Park Heritage Museum.)

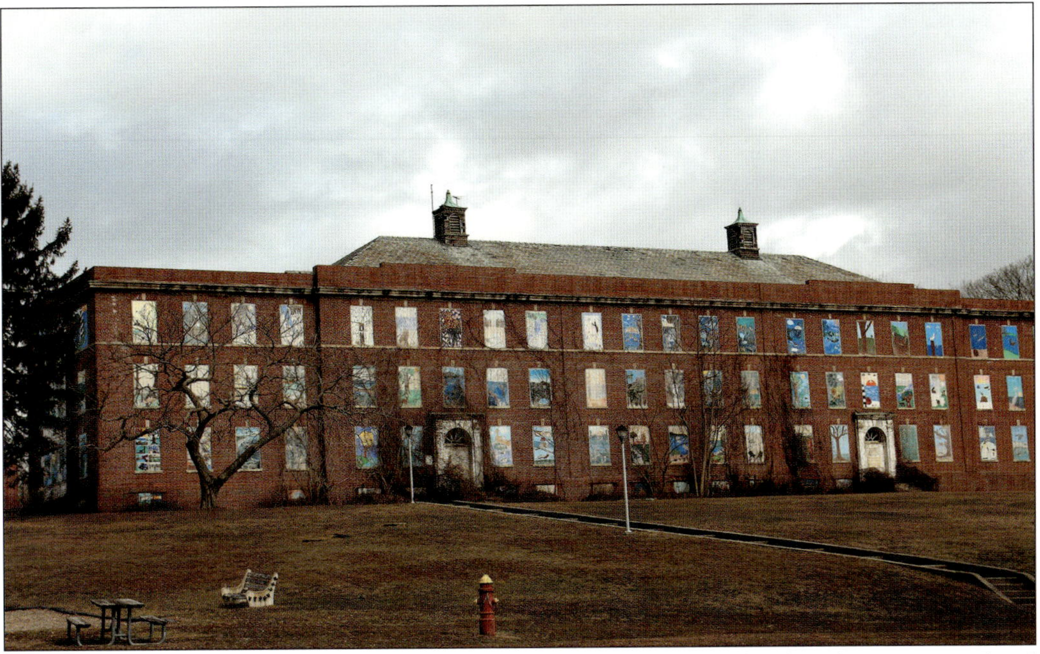

The brand-new employee home, which Dr. Macy had been instrumental in founding, was completed in 1919 and promptly named the Macy House in his honor. Macy, who died on May 22, 1918, led the hospital through the period of rapid growth. The former nurse's home was renamed the Dewey Home in memory of former superintendent Dr. Oliver Dewing.

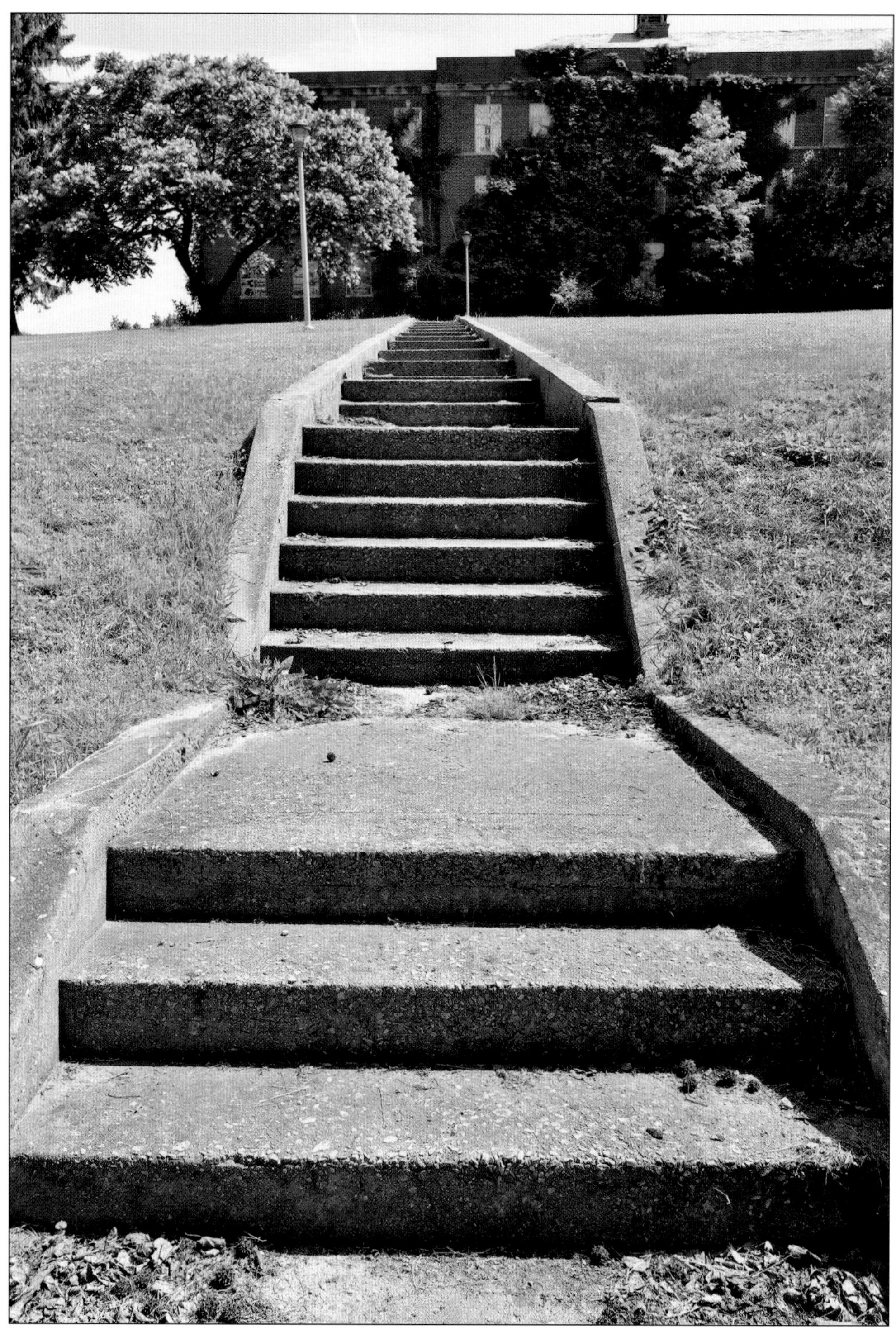

Also in 1919, the alumni association for the nursing school organized with a membership of 22 men and 75 women. The legislature authorized a 13 percent salary increase. The state, however, was unable to pay the higher rate because of loss of revenue due to Prohibition.

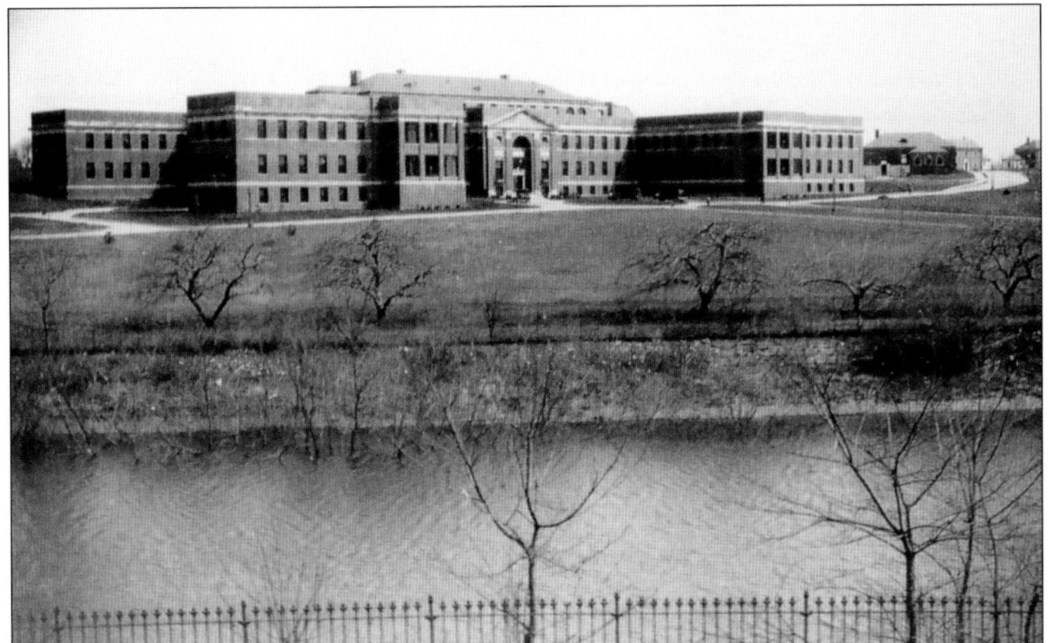

The salary increase was finally implemented in 1920. Simultaneously, the salary of female ward employees was raised to that of male employees. Even the return of employees from the military did not alleviate the staff shortages. There had been a mere 12 doctors for 4,479 patients. This photograph is of Building L. (Courtesy of the Leo P. Ostebo Kings Park Heritage Museum.)

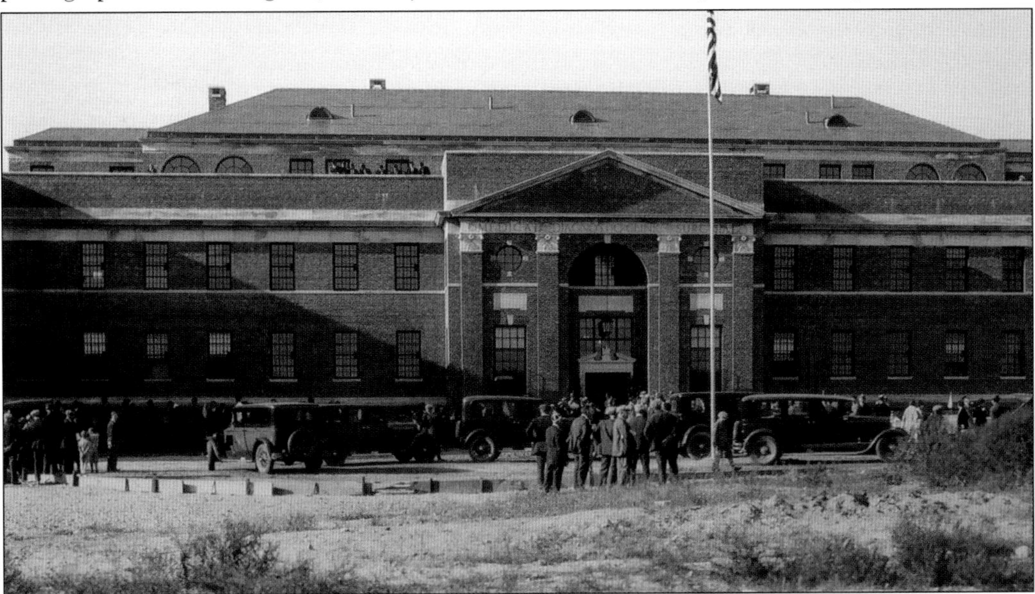

By 1920, the clinics were opening. There were strong recommendations to hold clinics at additional sites and to increase the hours, including some evenings. More and more patients were being placed on what was referred to as "parole." The social work staff was increased, and a physician, a secretary, and several attendants were detailed to oversee and develop the parole program. This photograph shows the Medical/Surgery/X-Ray/Laboratory Building. (Courtesy of the Leo P. Ostebo Kings Park Heritage Museum.)

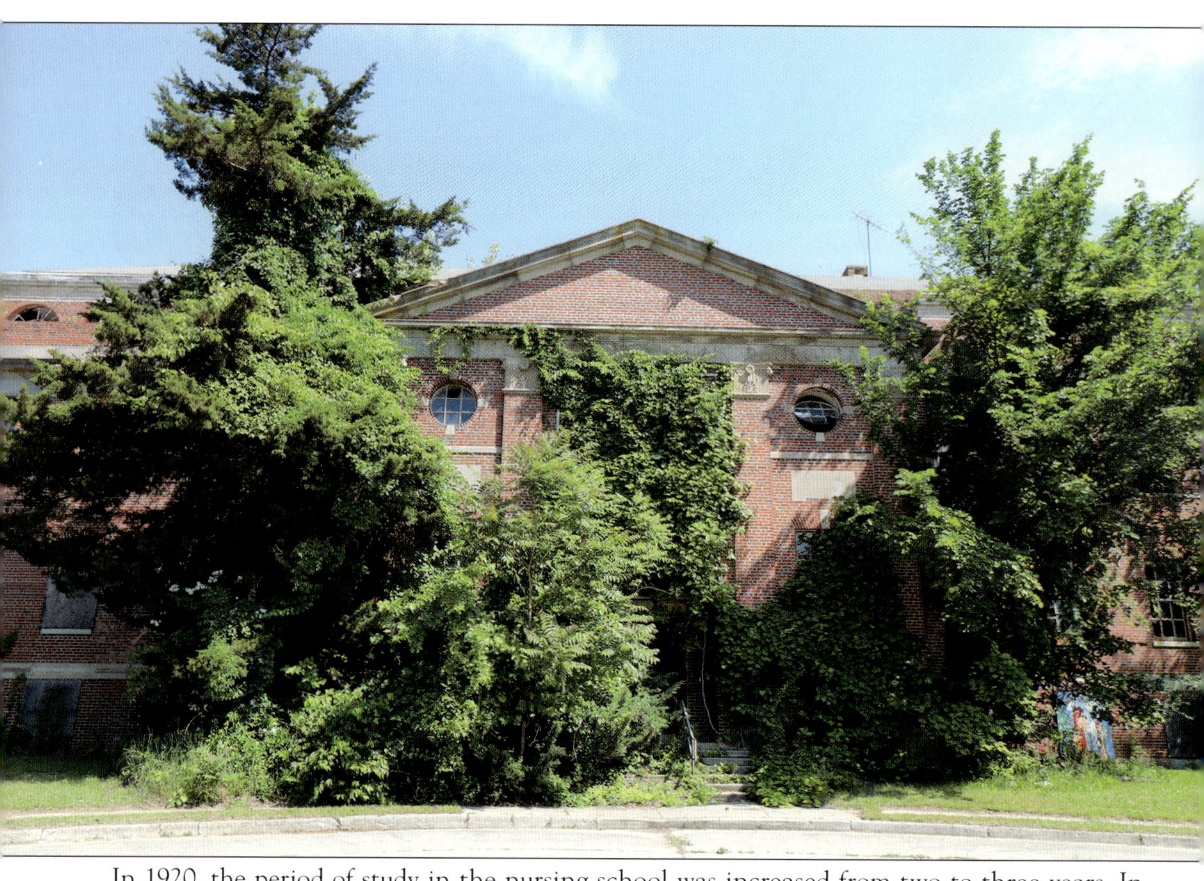

In 1920, the period of study in the nursing school was increased from two to three years. In 1923, the federal government began construction of a new group of buildings for veterans. This photograph shows the Medical/Surgery/X-Ray/Laboratory Building.

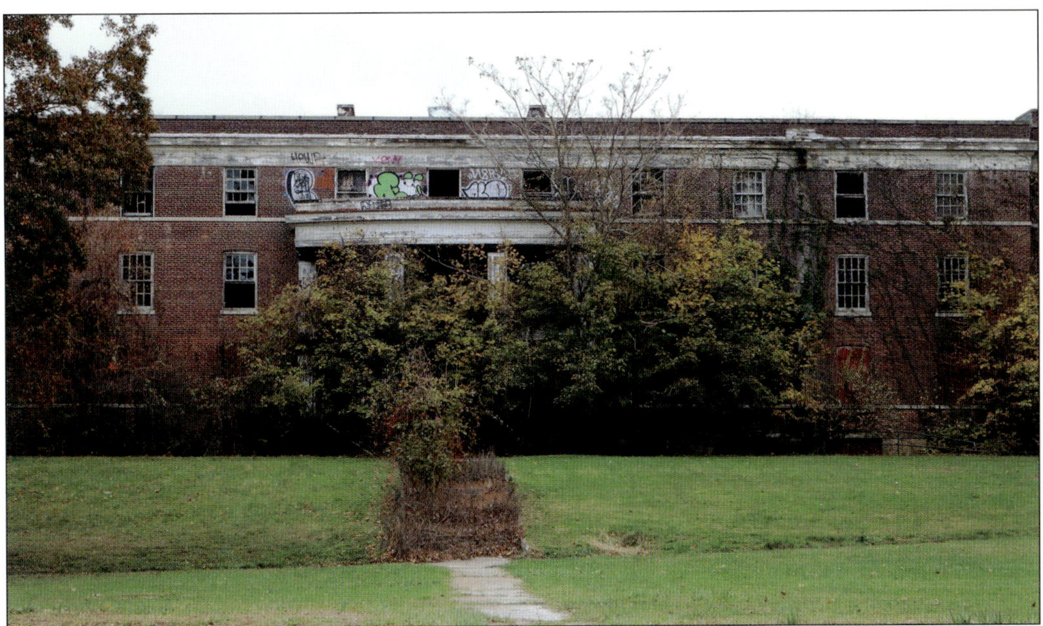

Wings were added to Macy House, and a kitchen and dining room were added. The Female Reception Building opened, as well as the Veterans' Memorial Hospital Unit. On July 4, 1923, Gov. Alfred E Smith oversaw the ground-breaking for the new reservoir, with a capacity 1,500,000 gallons. The lower reservoir was abandoned because of surface drainage; the upper reservoir was leaking. The following photographs are of Macy House.

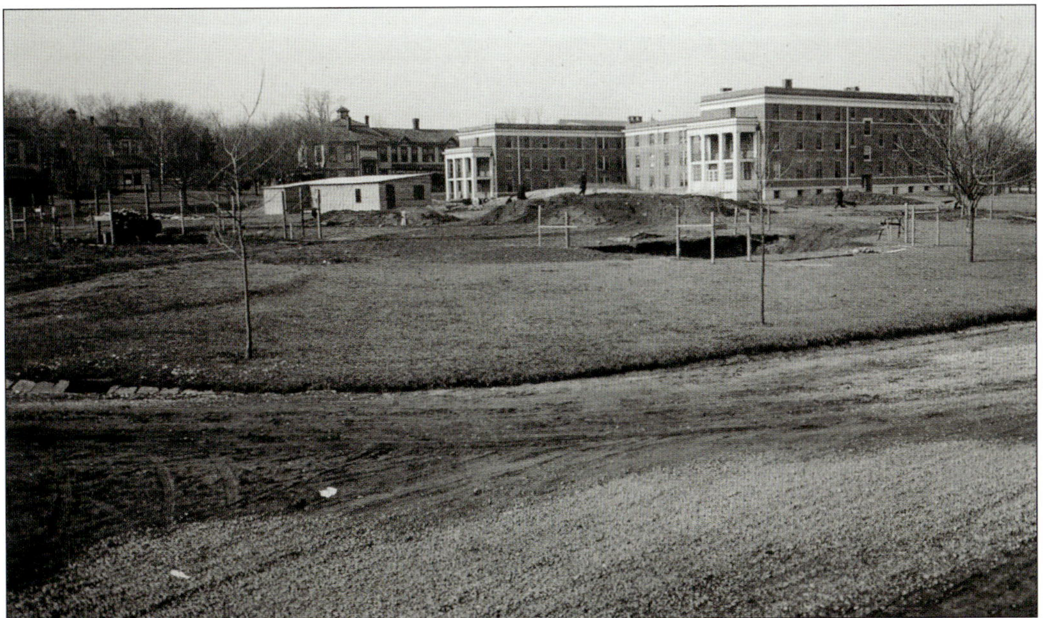

In 1926, construction continued. A new firehouse was built, along with more staff cottages and a children's ward, which was designed for boys under the age of 12. The Veterans' Memorial Hospital Unit, comprised of 17 new fireproof buildings, was dedicated on September 24, 1927. The unit was built by the federal government at a cost of $1 million. (Courtesy of the Leo P. Ostebo Kings Park Heritage Museum.)

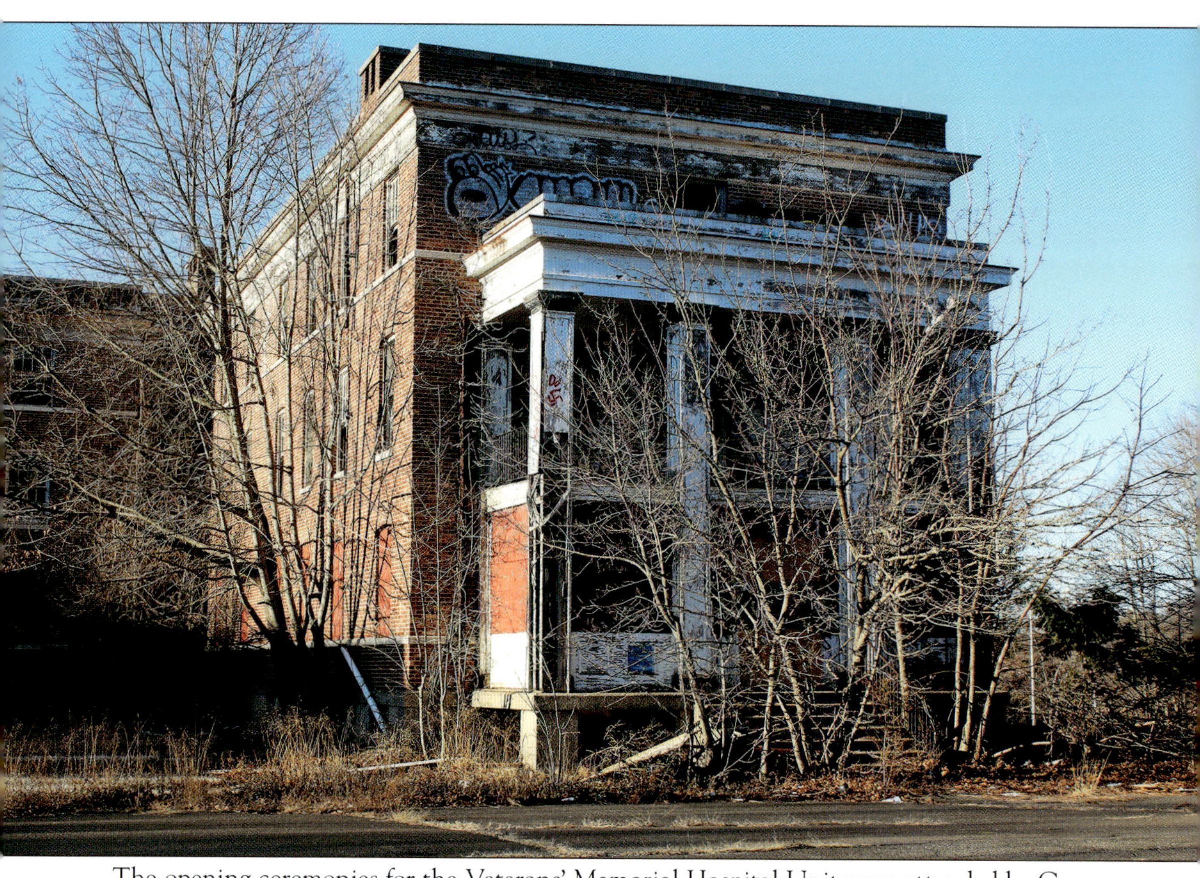

The opening ceremonies for the Veterans' Memorial Hospital Unit were attended by Governor Smith, along with many federal, state, and local dignitaries. This group of buildings was used to house war veterans in need of long-term psychiatric care.

Five

The 1920s through the Modern Day

The Kings Park hamlet was a "company town," but the company was not a traditional industry; it treated people who had problems coping with reality. A large proportion of town residents worked at the hospital. Kings Park was different from most state hospitals because of its combination of a waterfront site and complex topography. Its location provided beautiful vistas both toward and away from the hospital. The river is exceptionally wide within sight of Kings Park, and the sound is also wide yet narrow enough to see Connecticut. The land ranges from sea level to 250 feet, creating several scenic overlooks. KPSH was also different because of the people who worked there. The culture of the town was diverse, its people compassionate and determined to treat the patients of the hospital the best they could. They became family. It was not always this way. After the generations of the 1930s, 1940s, and 1950s passed on, new ideas came along with outsiders, and the way patients were treated for mental illness had begun to change—less therapy, more drugs. Less medical dispensing of the drugs led to less caretaking, assuming the patients would take the drugs on their own and purposefully lead productive lives. However, mental illness does not always work that way. Once the hospital closed, like many of the mental hospitals at the time, patients were mostly left with no one to care for them and left to fend for themselves. There was a reason they were in a hospital in the first place. There are very few places today dedicated to the mentally ill, yet mental illness has not gone away.

—David Flynn

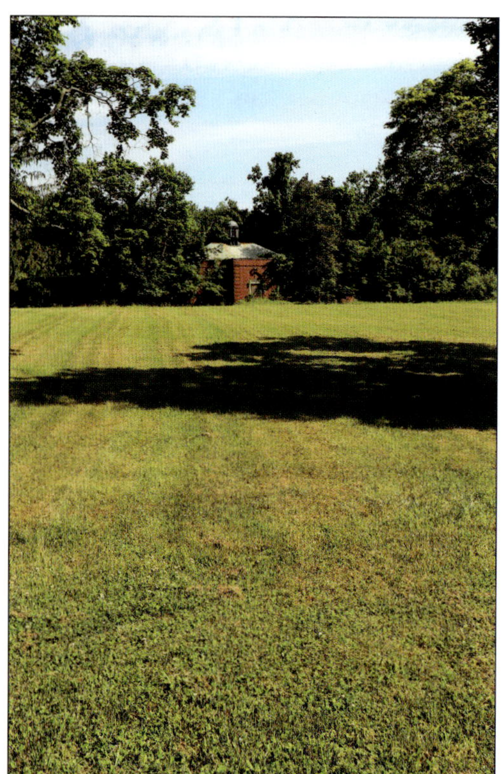

One of the ways the facility kept patients busy and brought in some revenue was a thriving business of manufacturing wicker furniture and baskets. Patients and workers planted groves of willow trees, called holts, which in 1928 yielded 850 pounds of willow. The following photographs are of the Mental Retardation Unit.

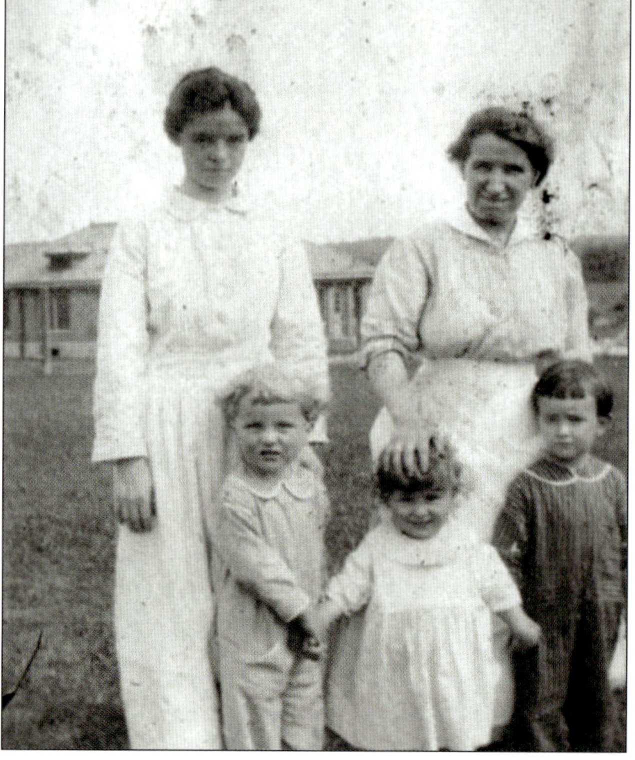

The 1920s and 1930s saw very active treatment services for syphilis. The clinic was in session three times a week. The drugs neoarsphenamine, tryparsamide, and mercury including bismuth were used, as was hyperthermia using malaria or typhoid. (Courtesy of the Leo P. Ostebo Kings Park Heritage Museum.)

A new laboratory building was completed in 1930. The following year, the facility expanded its clinical services. This dramatic expansion included extended care at Cumberland Hospital in Brooklyn, the Mineola Red Cross building, and Huntington and Riverhead and a monthly child guidance clinic.

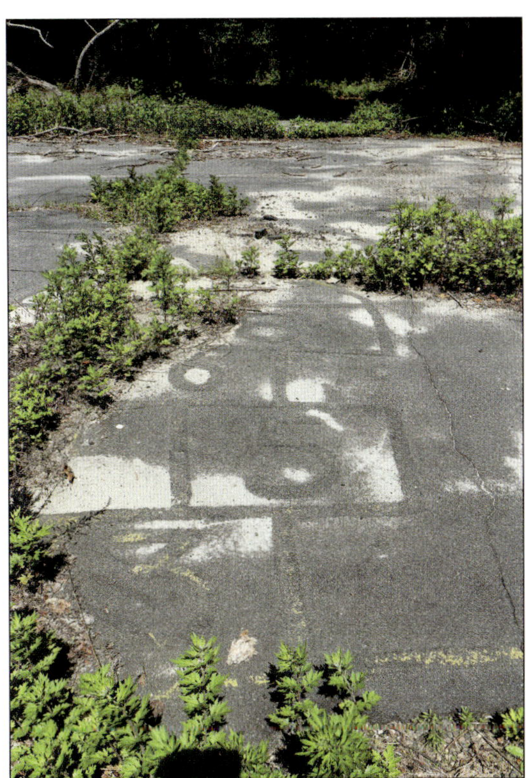

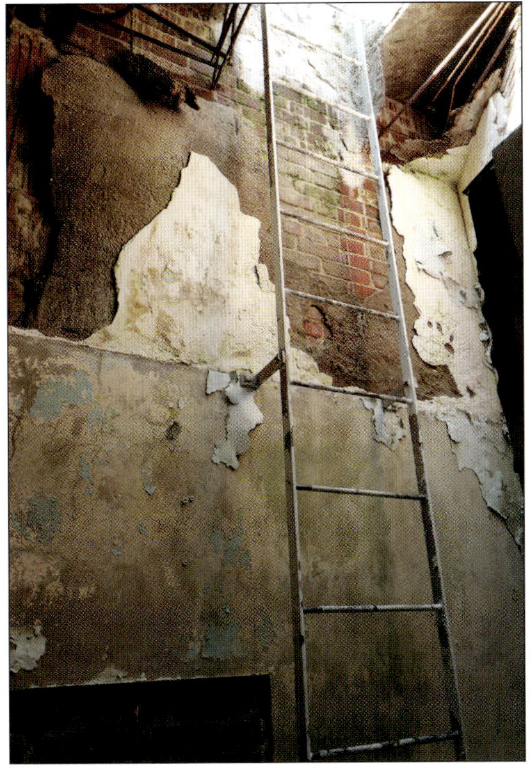

There were also plans to take over clinics that been held sporadically at Greenport, Freeport, Oyster Bay, Glen Cove, Great Neck, and Nantucket, Rhode Island.

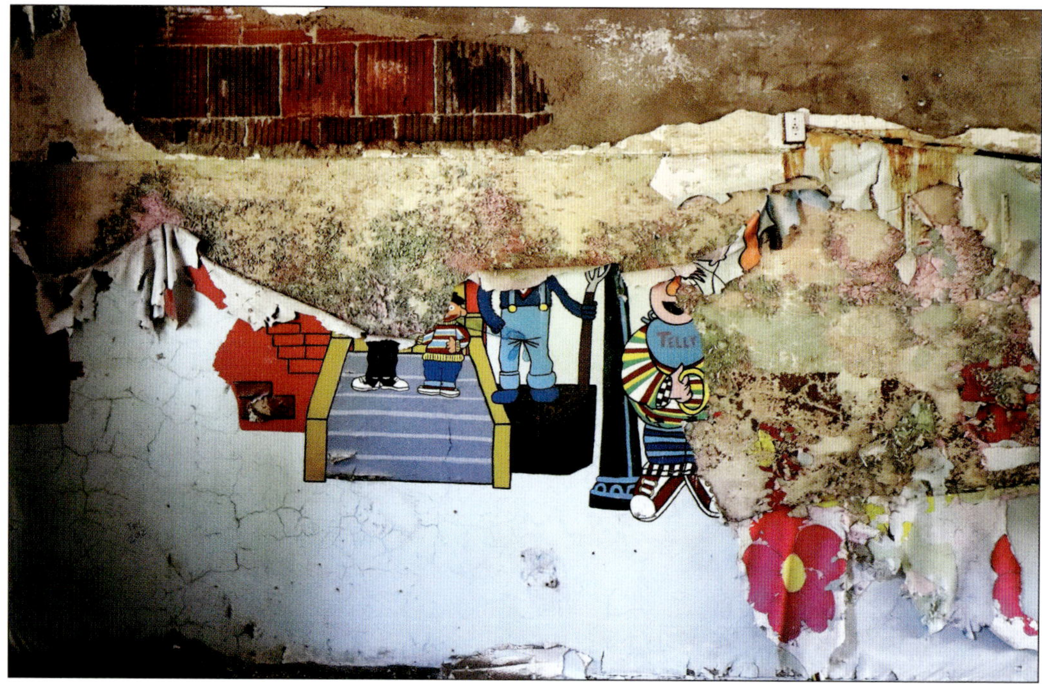

In 1931, though the maximum capacity was set at 3,712, the actual patient count was at 5,775. In hopes of alleviating the overcrowding, patients were transferred to upstate hospitals: 100 to Esther and 500 to Mercy.

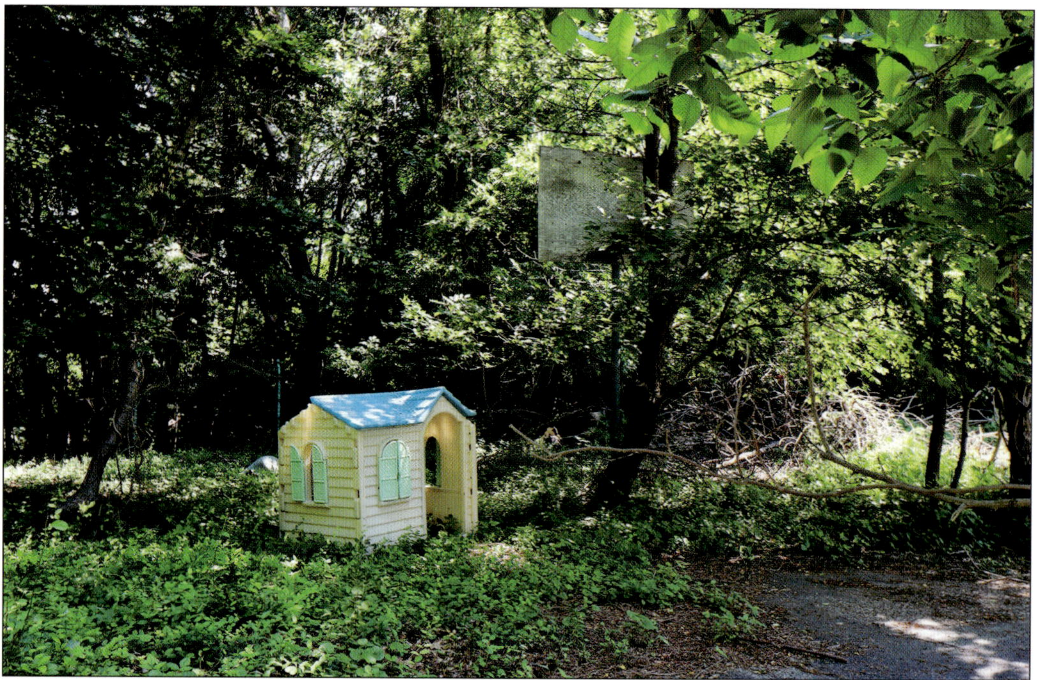

In 1932, Pilgrim State Hospital opened in Brentwood to alleviate overcrowded conditions at Kings Park and Central Islip. On September 7, 1932, the brand-new York Hall was officially dedicated.

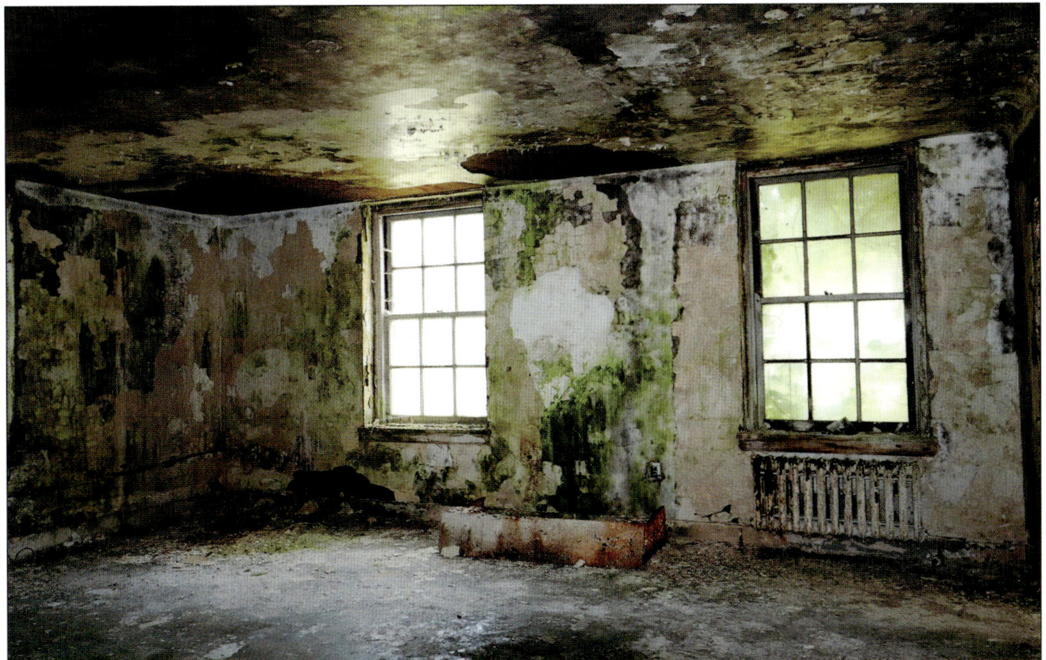

The first religious service held there, however, was on Sunday, May 22. At the official dedication, the facility was named in honor of Monsignor John C. York. Father York had long been the secretary of the board of visitors and had been instrumental in securing funds to build the hall.

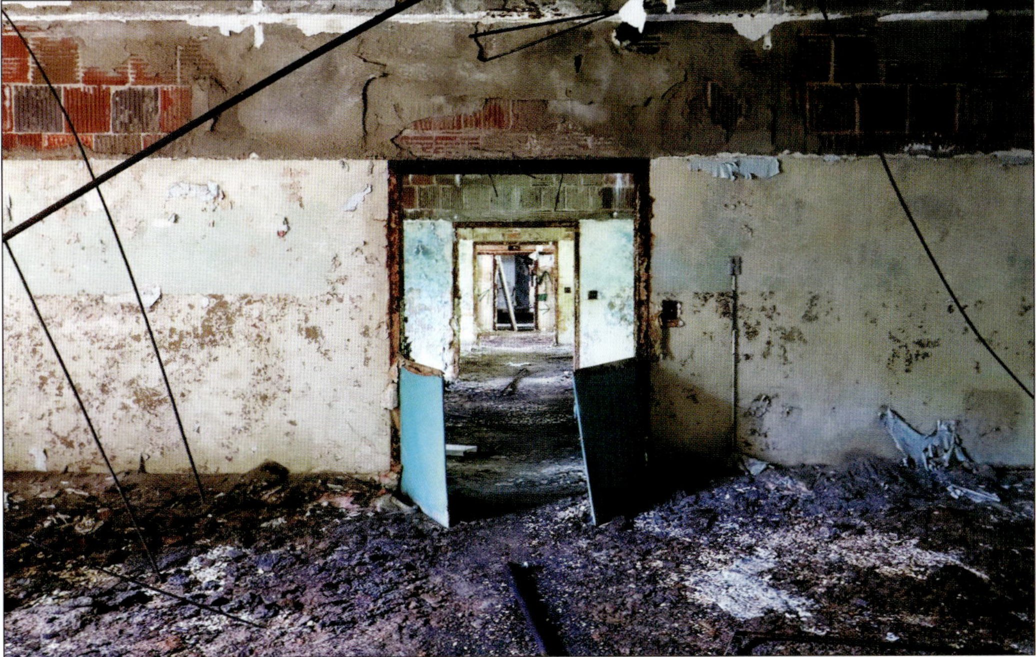

Pilgrim Psychiatric Center, the world's largest psychiatric center at the time, was opened in 1932. Dr. William Tiffany, the superintendent of Kings Park, was transferred there, as were large numbers of patients. An athletic field was dedicated to Dr. Tiffany on June 9, 1934. Kings Park Tiffany Field remains popular.

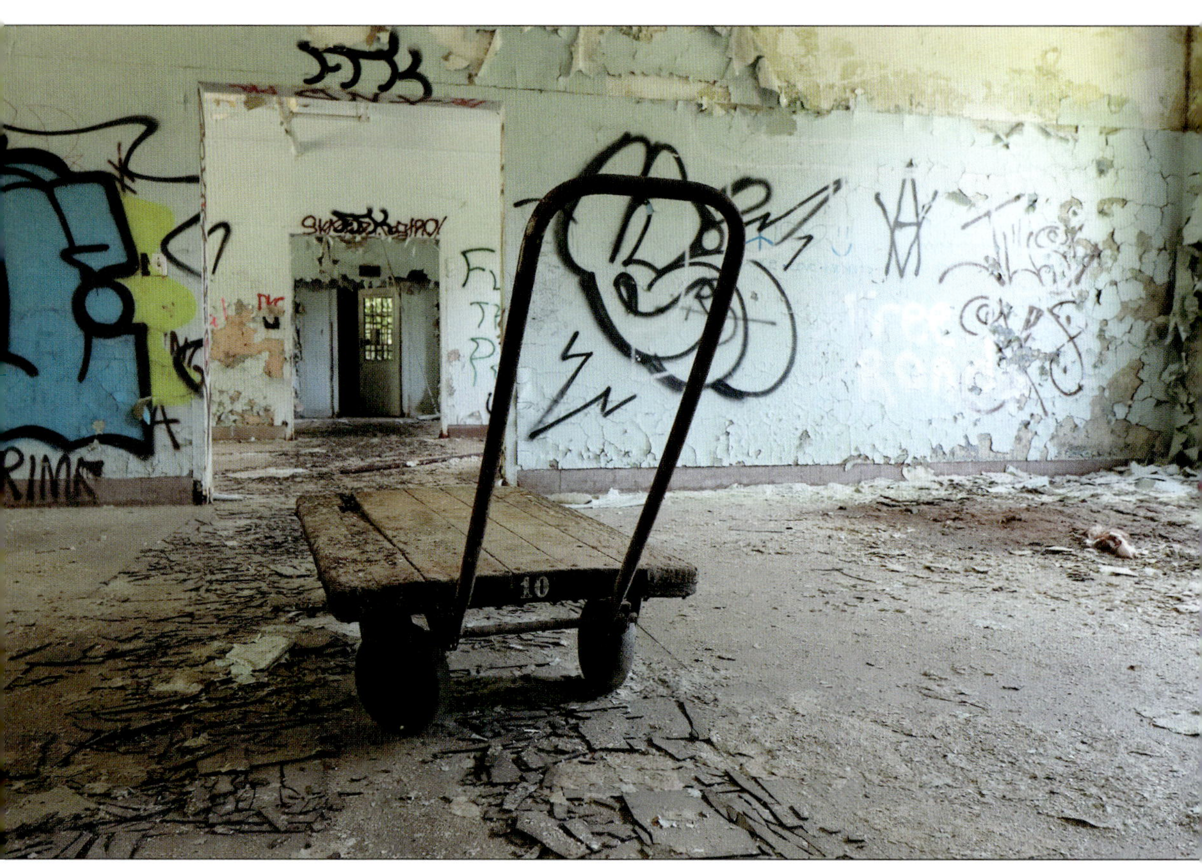

Construction continued throughout the 1930s. In 1933, the new operating center for the acute and surgical wards was added to Building L, Veterans' Memorial Hospital. It provided an operating room suite and wards for the care of medical and surgical patients from all parts of the hospital. It also included an employees' infirmary.

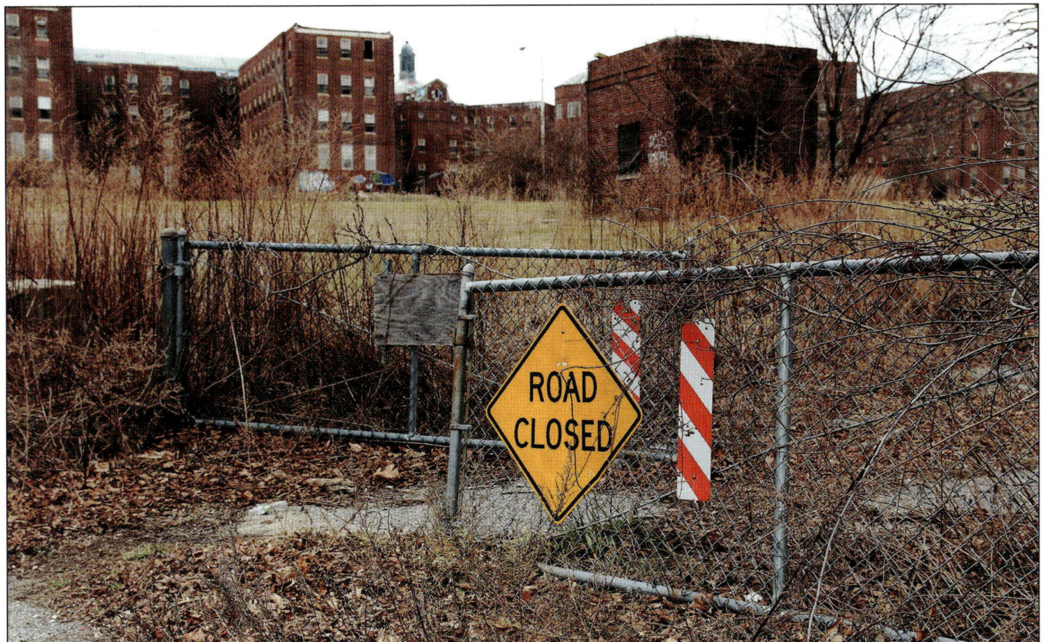

The following year, Building L, also known as the Veterans' Group, became the first stand-alone medical surgical center for patients and employees. Prior to this, the medical unit was located in a patient building. Patients coming from the city for admission had been transported in special compartments and/or cars on the Long Island Rail Road. This practice was discontinued in 1936, when buses were provided for that purpose.

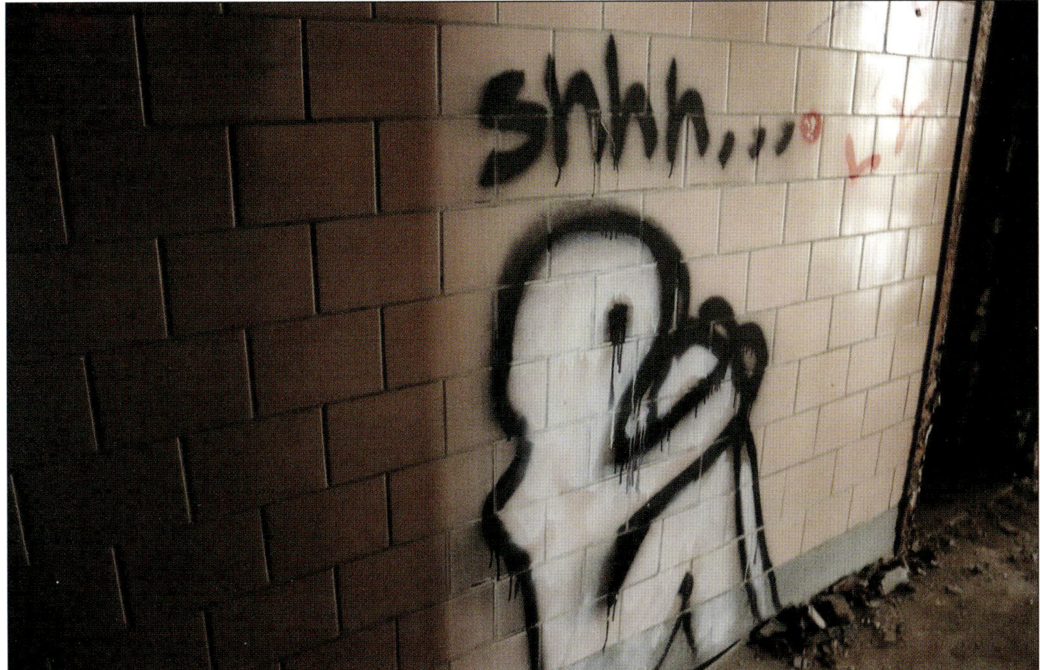

In 1935, the capacity of the institution was set at 4,086; the actual number of patients, however, was 5,019 (minus 526 who had been placed on parole). Shown here is the Administration Building.

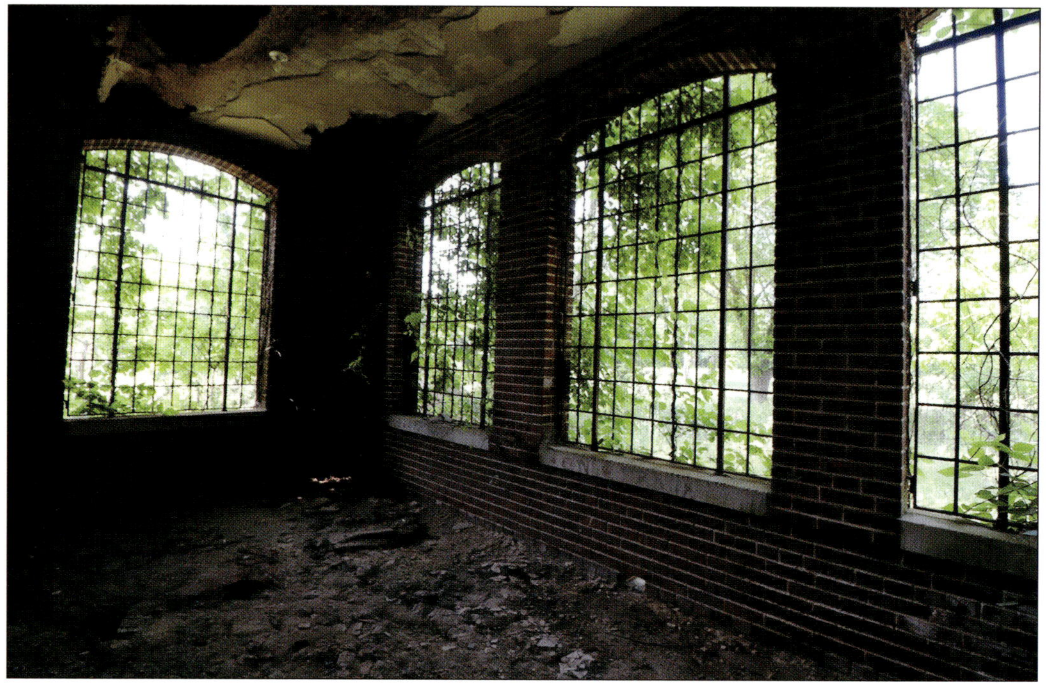

There were 34 on the medical staff, three dentists, and 34 nonmedical staff. Of the graduates of the nursing school, 21 men and 70 women were employed. Ward attendants included 269 men and 139 women. This photograph is of the Mental Retardation Unit.

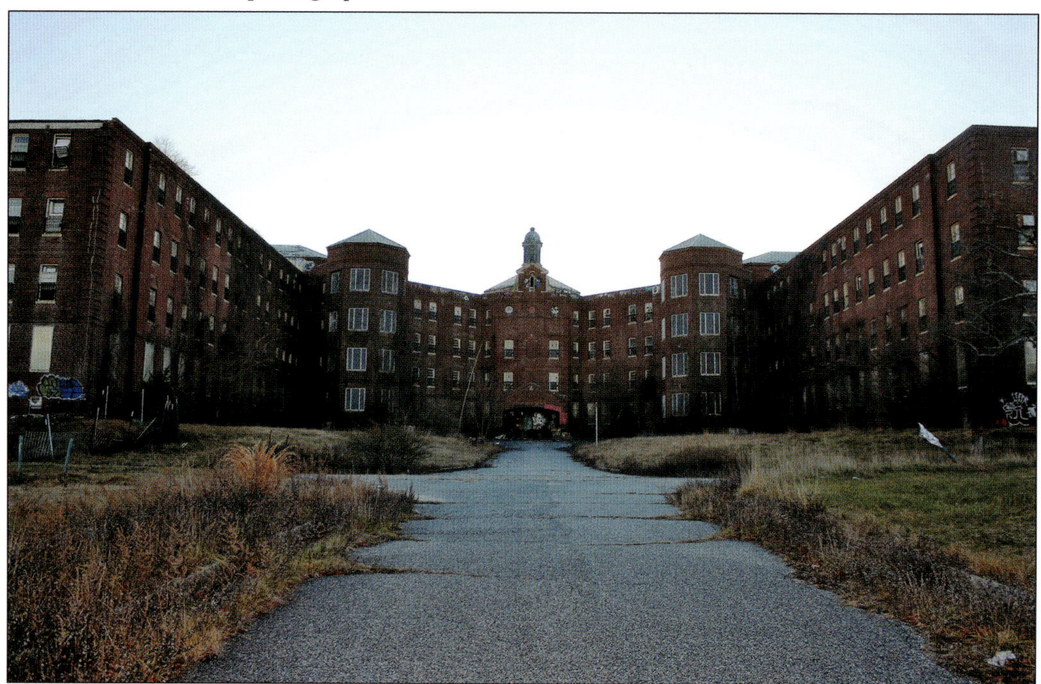

On March 1, 1936, the nursing school expanded to include students from general hospitals. These trainees spent three months of instruction in the care of the mentally ill. Shown here are Wards 101–128, which housed the kitchen and dining room.

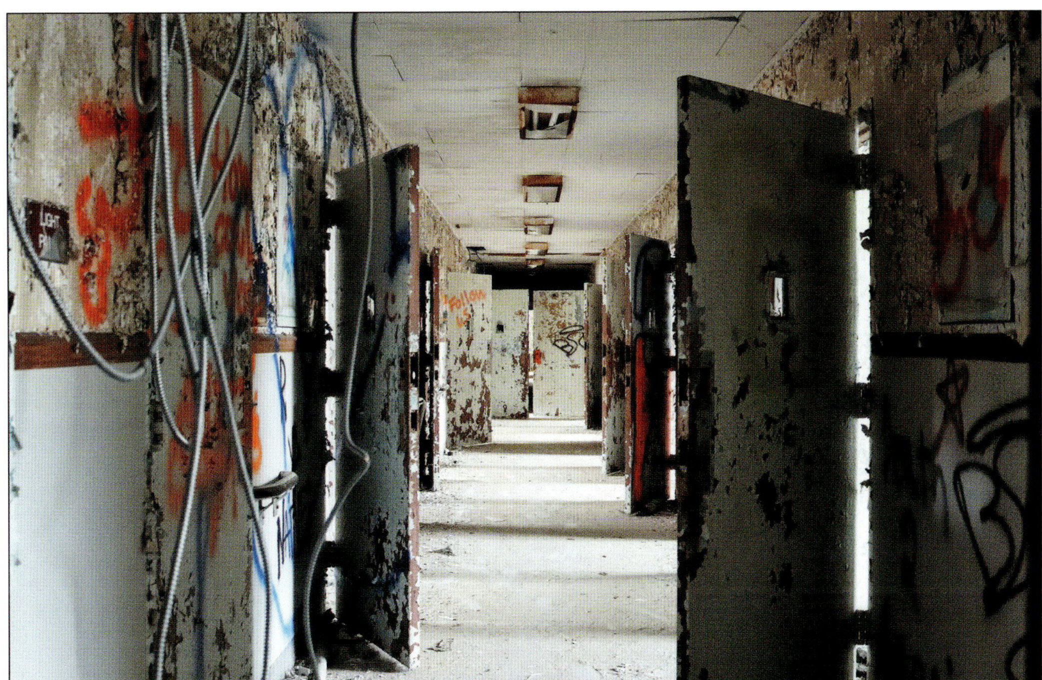

The same year saw the addition of wards set aside for convulsive therapy for patients with schizophrenia. The technique used was insulin therapy. By 1948, the shock therapy department occupied the third floor of Building 93 and treated 638 patients—439 with electroshock, 118 with insulin, and 111 with a combination of both. Shown here is the Mental Retardation Unit.

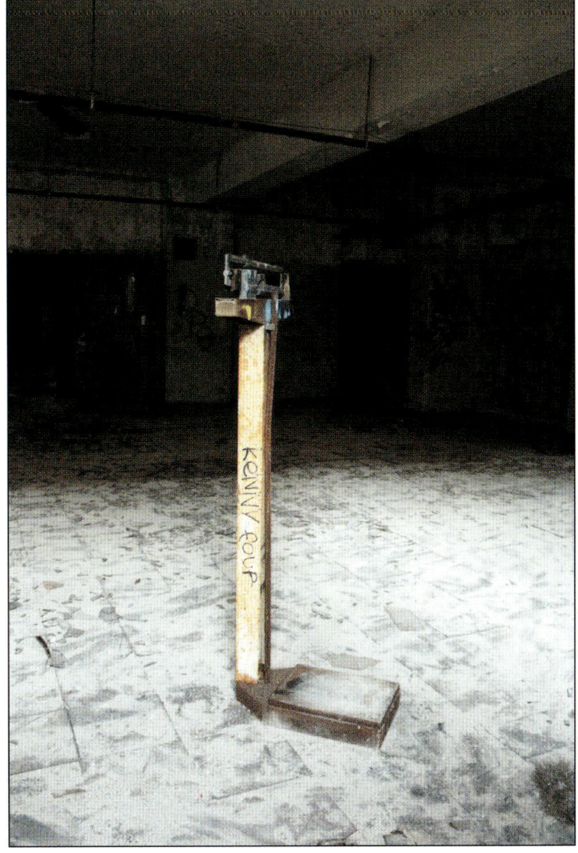

Kings Park was composed of a group of cottages meant to avoid the high-rise asylum model, which was already viewed as inhumane. But with psychiatric hospitals well over capacity in New York City into the 1930s, in 1939, the institution began constriction of Building 93, a 13-story structure. The following photographs show wards 101–128, which housed the kitchen and dining room.

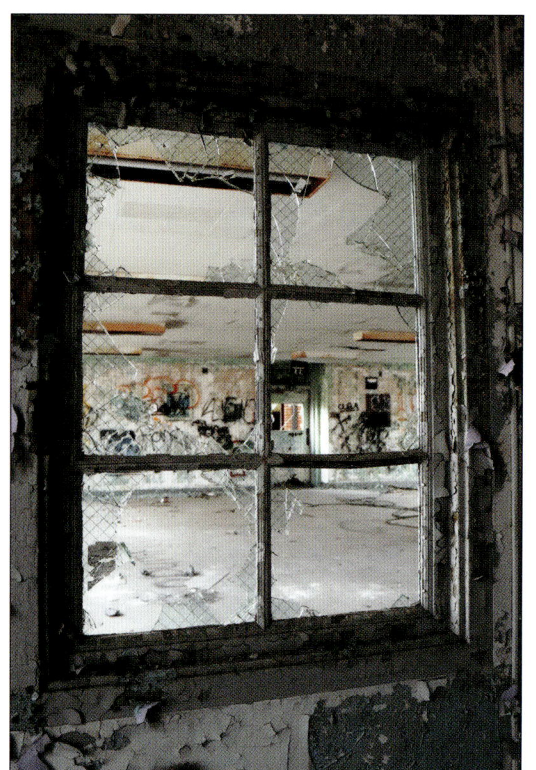

At its peak in the 1950s, Kings Park reached a population of over 10,000 residents, who were divided by gender, age, temperament, and physical limitations through a complex of over 100 buildings, which included power plants, fire stations, staff housing, hospitals, recreational facilities, piggeries, and cow barns.

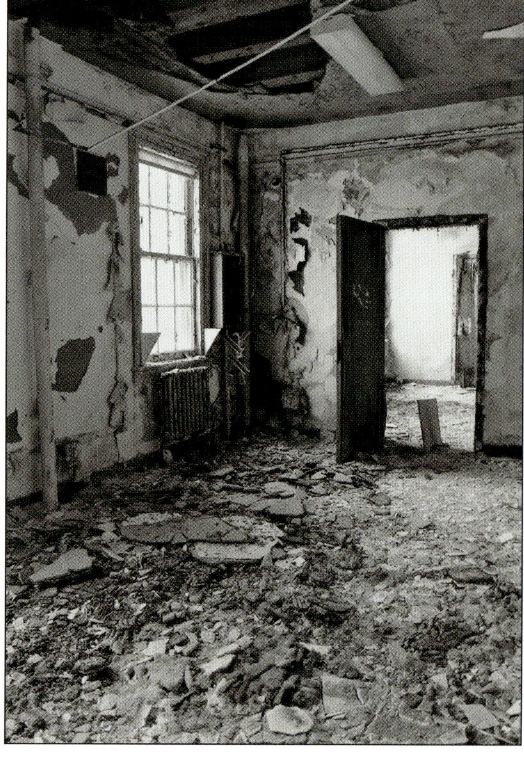

By 1940, construction of Building 93 was completed, along with the superintendent's residence, a seven-family staff house, and a five-family staff house. The nursing school had 465 graduates in April of that year. The Psych Center had also expanded its services to include group therapy in 1944.

In 1947, the recreation department was established in New York state hospitals. This brought the first television set to the facility, which was installed on Ward 85. In 1948, the patient count was 8,538. The veterans' division alone had 1,748, of which 832 were veterans of World War II, 890 from World War I, and 26 from the Spanish-American War. Shown here are Wards 17–38.

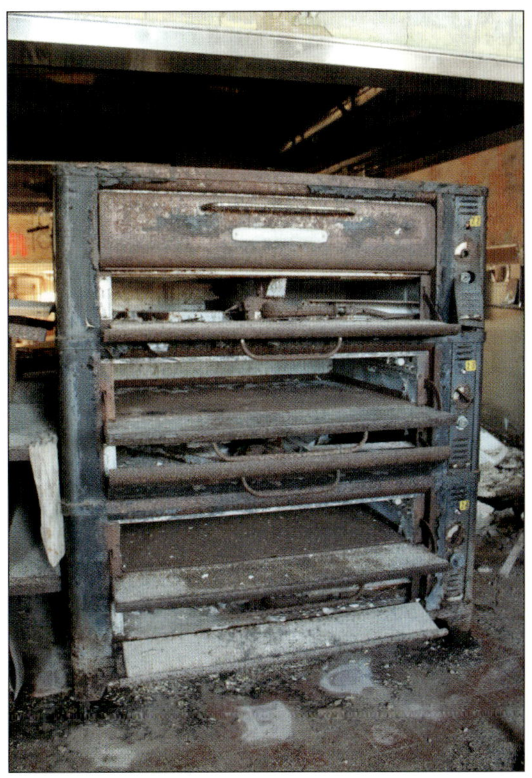

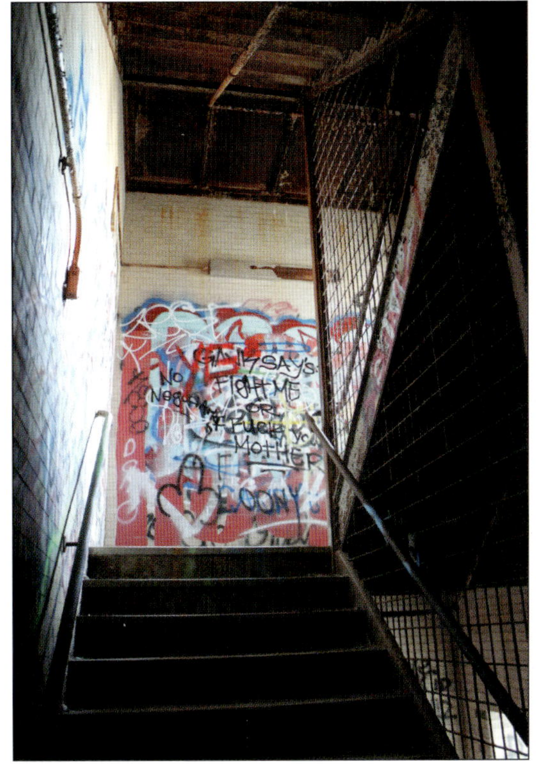

In January 1949, a large fire destroyed all of the industrial shops. Thankfully, there were no reports of injuries or fatalities. By March 1951, the patient count had reached 10,246, with a certified capacity of only 6,527. Shown here are Wards 101–128.

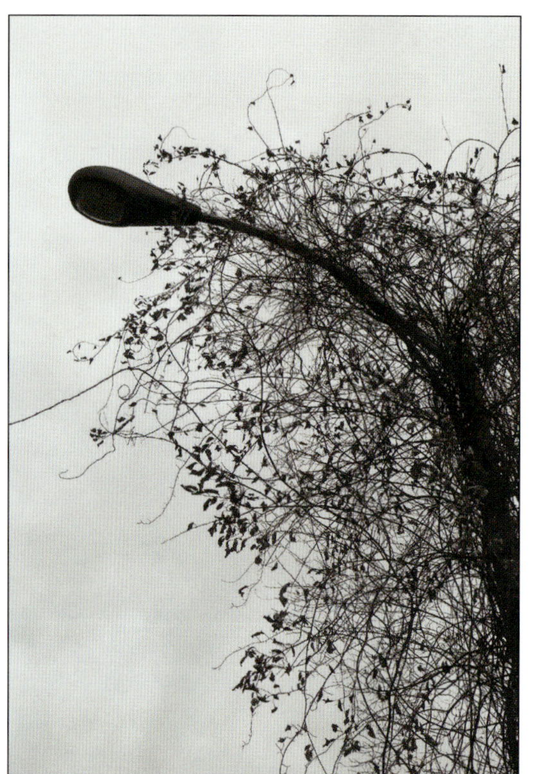

In December 1951, Dr. Meyer Rosenberg started doing prefrontal lobotomies on selected female patients, at the rate of two each week. In 1952, Dr. Charles Buckman was appointed senior director. A separate Children's Unit was organized on February 1, 1953. The children were separated by age groups, and special staff was provided for them. School classes were set up, and special occupational and recreational programs were devised.

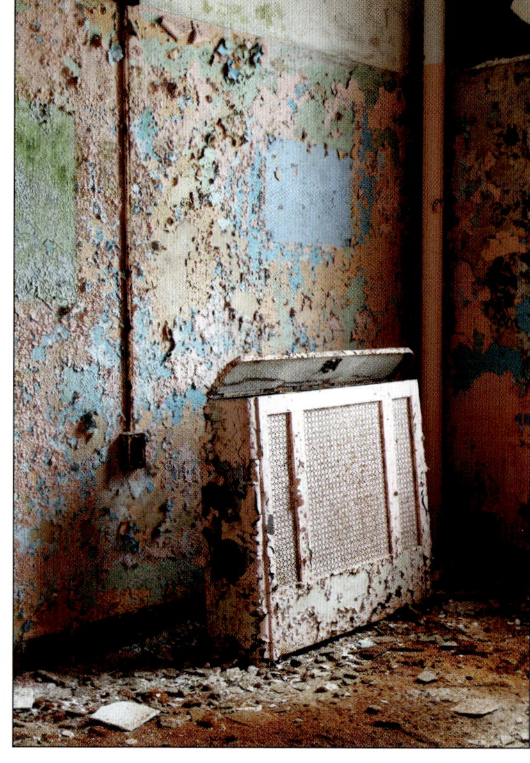

In 1953, ground was broken for a new laundry and a Physiotherapy Unit was formed. In August 1953, a physical therapist was appointed, and a physical therapy department opened in the basement of Building L. The mid-1950s brought the development of effective antipsychotic medications—and the end of extreme measures such as lobotomies and convulsive treatments.

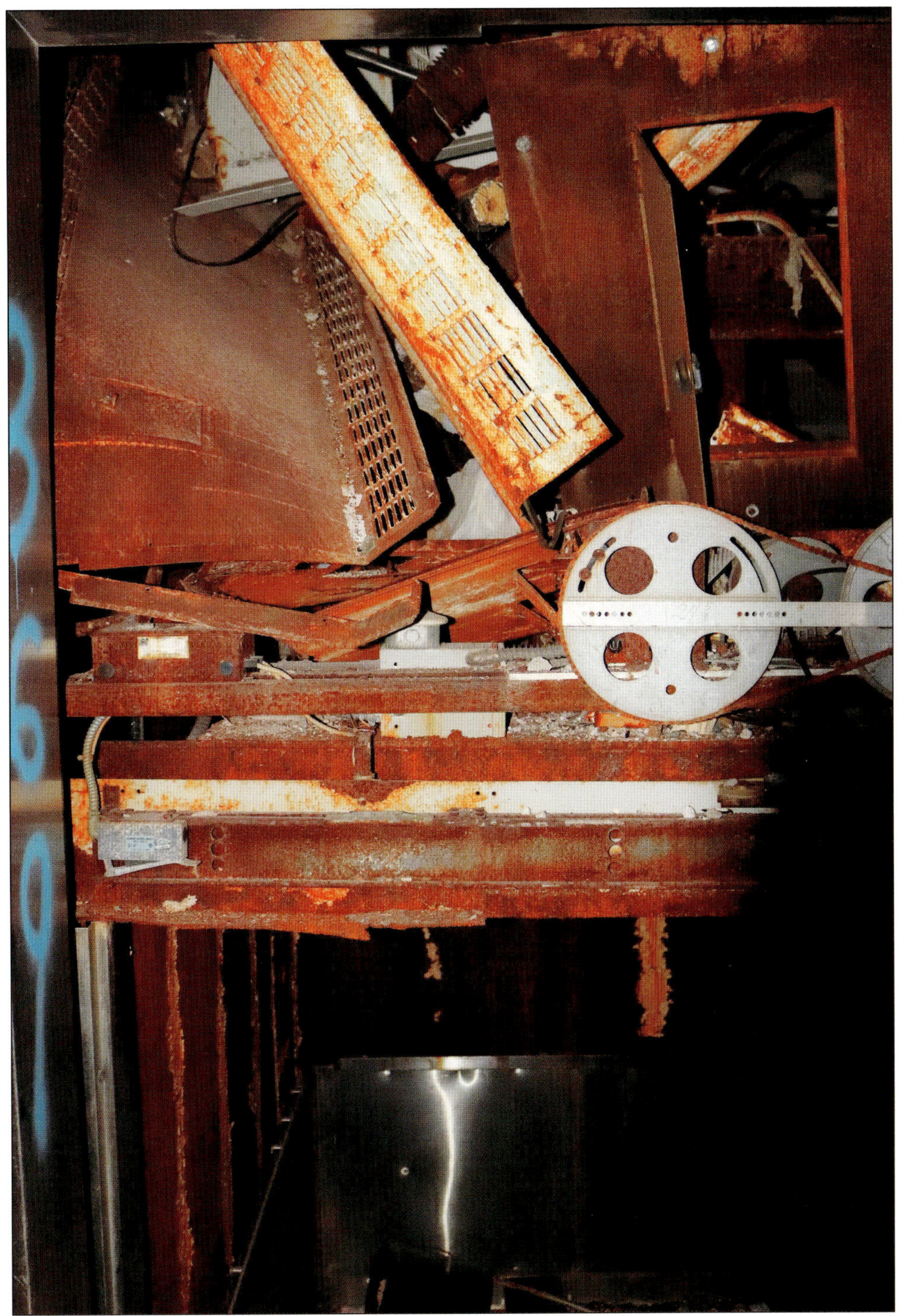

Use of Thorazine and Serpasil on an experimental basis was initiated in the fall of 1954. By the end of March 1955, some five percent of the patient population was receiving some sort of psychotropic drug therapy. The use of restraints declined by 50 percent. Psychosurgery was also declining. Shown here is the Medical/Surgery/X-Ray/Laboratory Building.

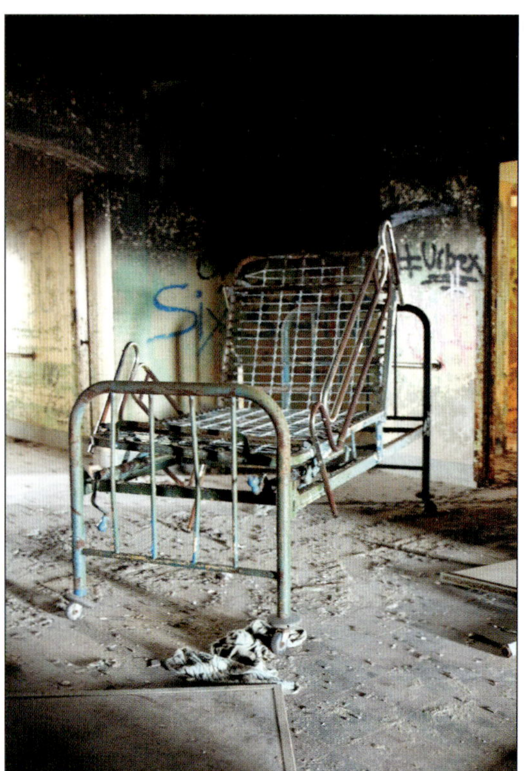

Thus began the declining need for such large facilities and barbaric treatments. For the first time, patients who had once been considered hopeless were able to manage their mental illness and live independently. Outpatient clinics were becoming more common, although some patients fell through the cracks nationwide. Shown here are Wards 101–128, which housed the kitchen and dining room.

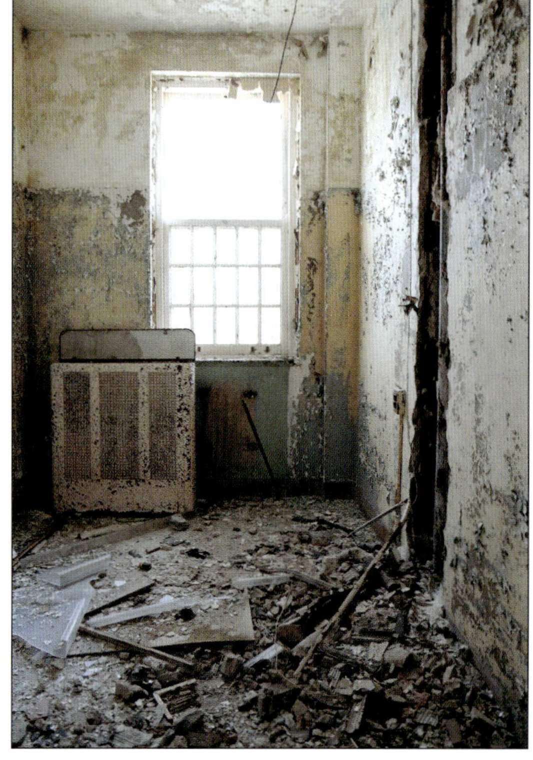

The introduction of medications led to a dramatic shift in institutions across the country from severe overcrowding to near abandonment. From the 1960s through the 1990s, deinstitutionalization swept through America. The unfortunate side effect, felt throughout the country, was that many patients who had lived in these facilities most of their lives were now on the street.

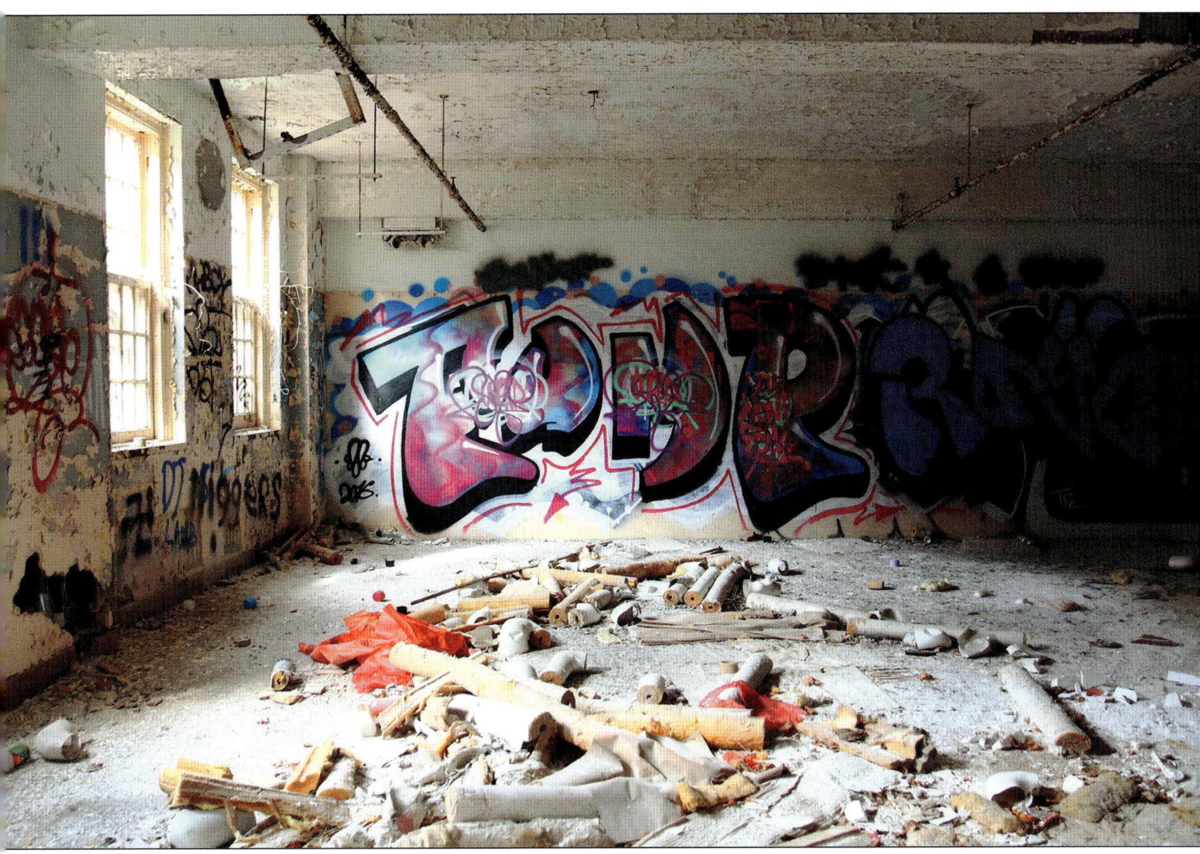

While the powers that be looked to put these types of facilities in the past, those who had known nothing else were left to fend for themselves. While some were helped by the new medications, others were not. Those who were helped still needed to remain compliant with their medication regime, and they often needed support in order to do so. This led to former patients living on the streets or incarcerated, without proper access to quality psychiatric care.

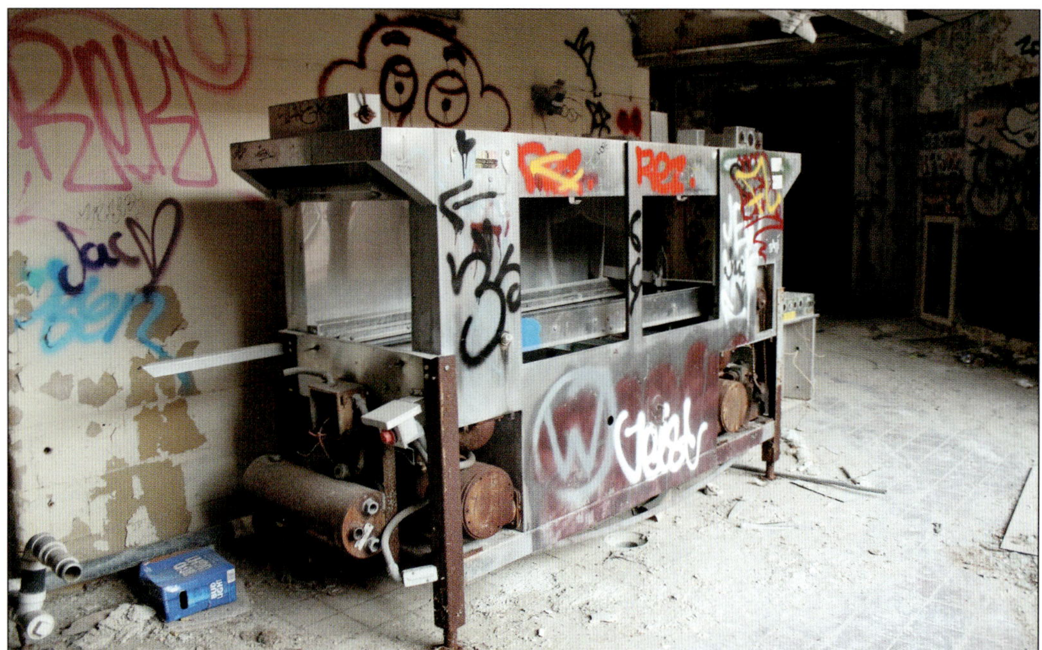

Building L was transitioned from the Veterans' Unit and became an independent medical surgical unit. In 1954, the hospital started Thorazine as an experimental treatment of mental illness. The following year, five percent of patients were on psychotropic drugs, and the use of restraints was down by half.

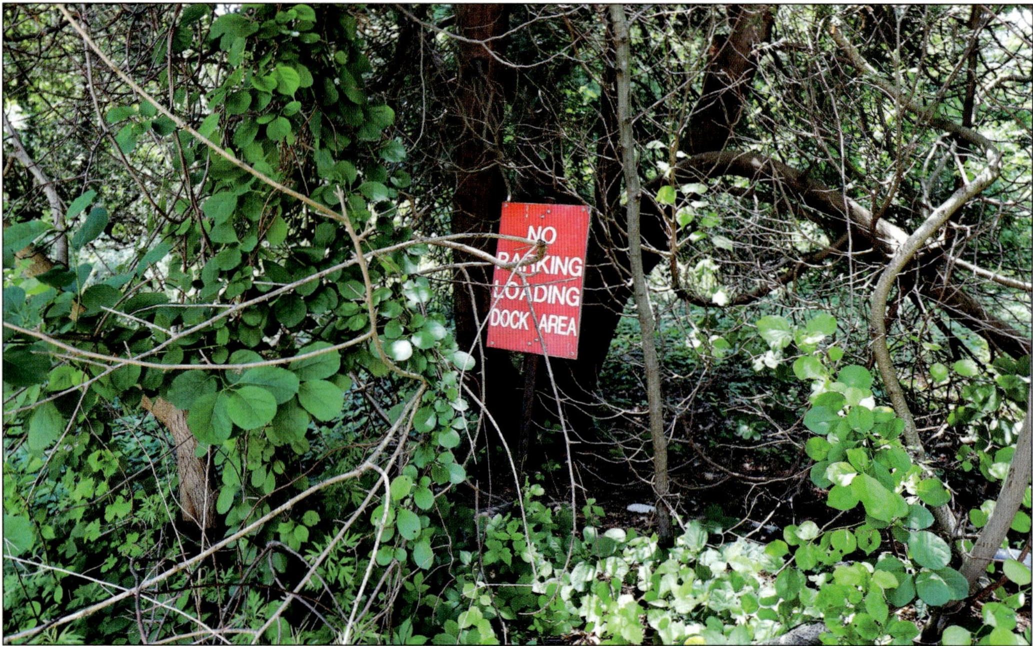

In 1955, the State of New York, feeling the financial burden of running mental health facilities, enacted the Mental Health Study Act. This called for the banishment of state-funded hospitals in favor of opening community centers to assist those with mental illness, which could be federally funded. The following photographs show Wards 81–84.

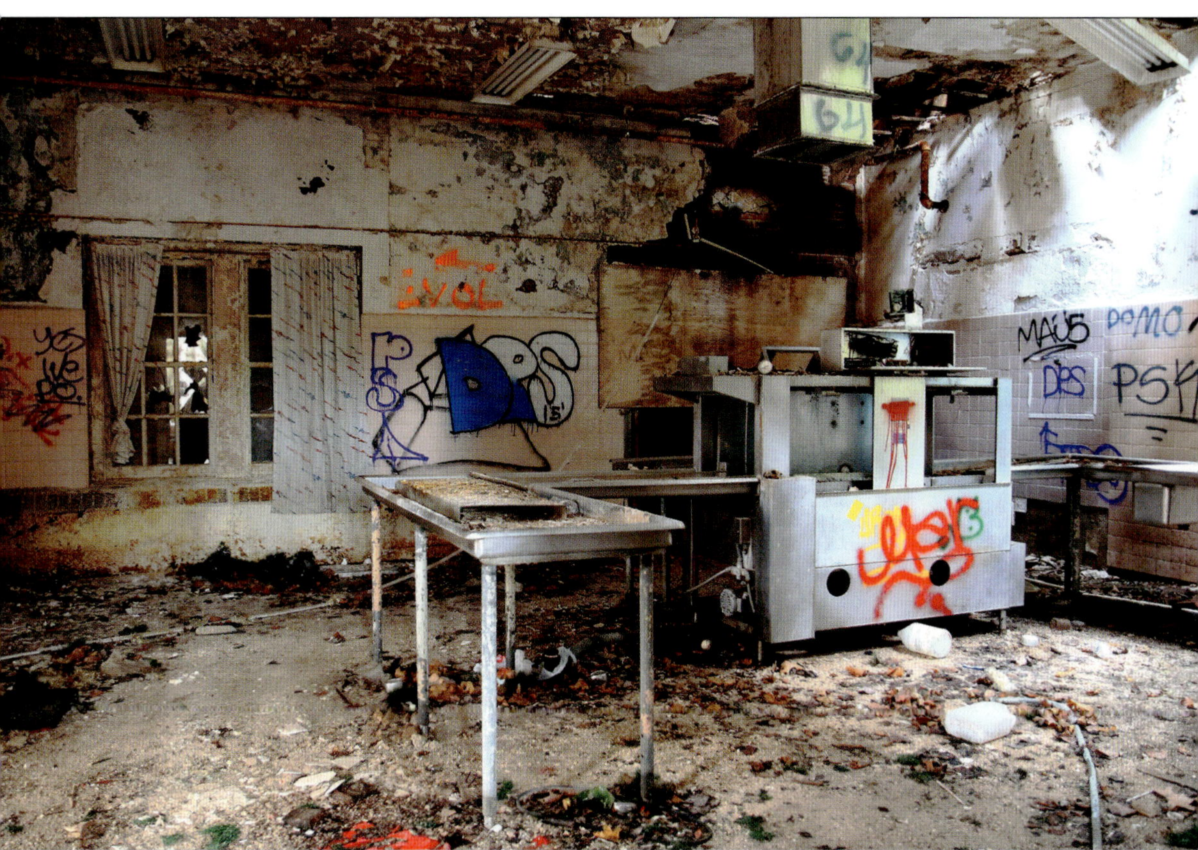

The farm, which had been such a prevalent feature on the hospital grounds, was phased out in the 1950s. It had become less expensive to buy the food, and the emphasis on work therapy had also waned. By 1965, nearly 100 acres had been sold off and 767 remained.

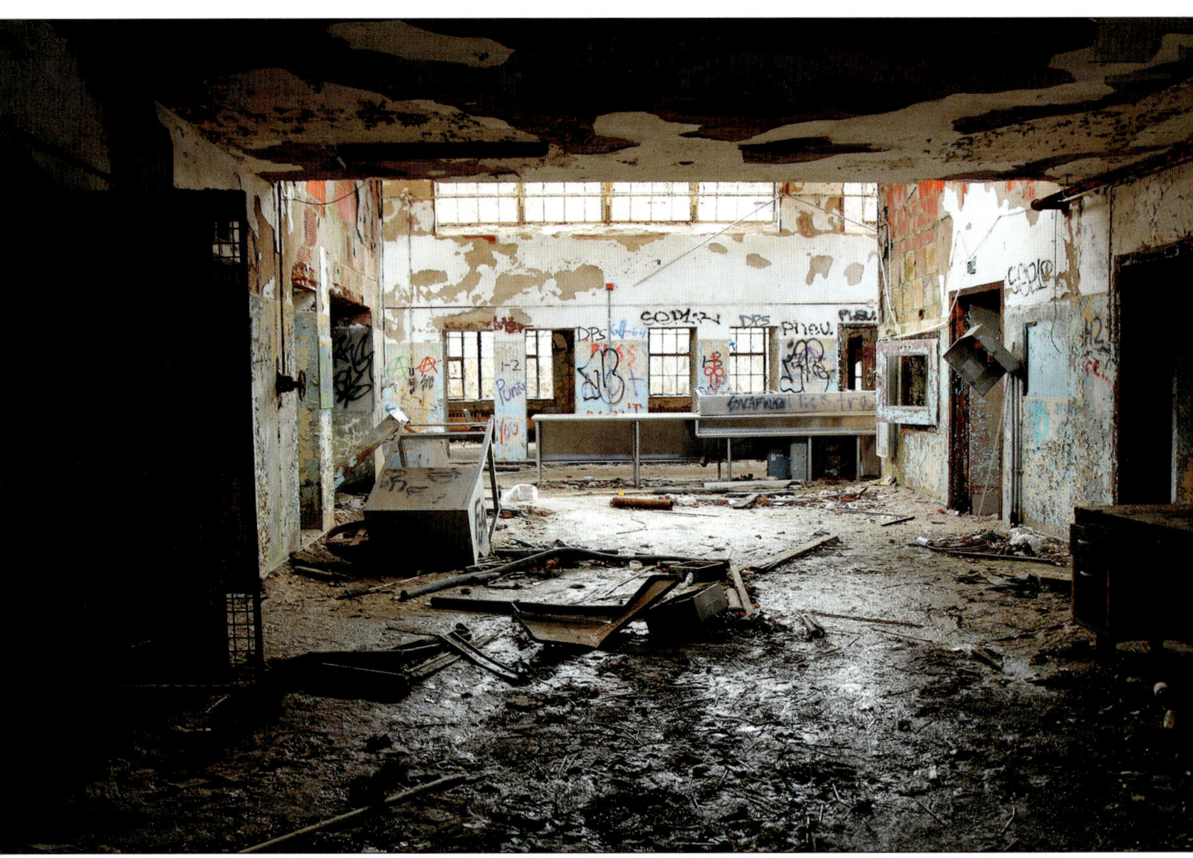

The nursing school had switched its affiliation from Kings Park to Huntington Hospital. Now, students were in residence at Kings Park throughout the three-year program. More time was available for scheduling classes, and the program was much easier to administer. In 1967, amid the expansive closures of state facilities, three buildings were opened: Building 21 as an administration service, Building 22 for children, and Building 7 for medicine and surgery.

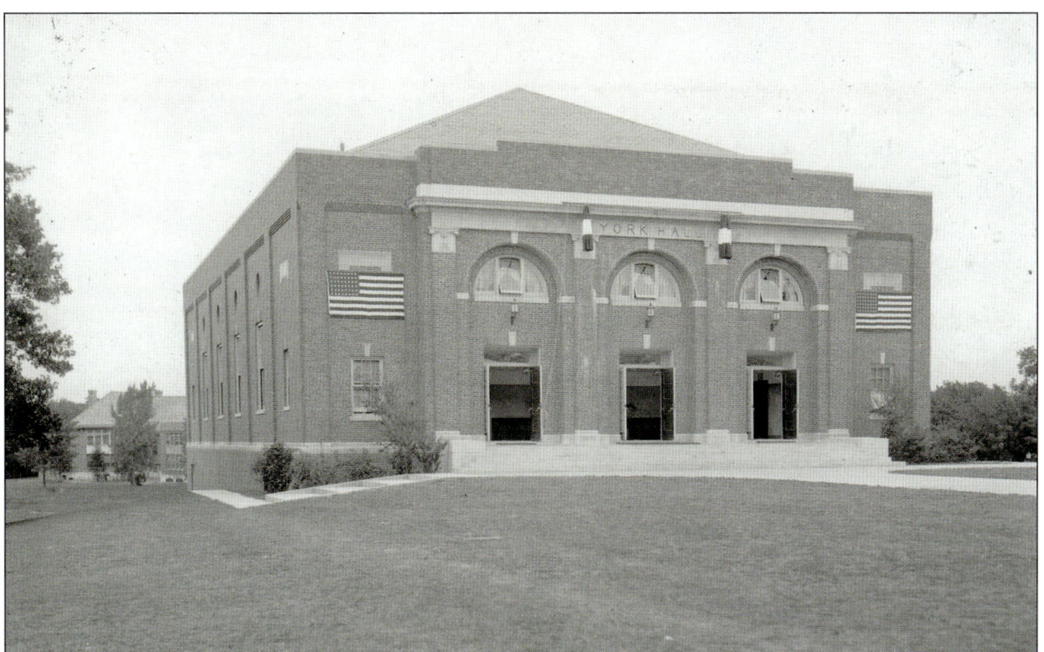

From the mid-1960s onward, the issues associated with deinstitutionalization became more apparent. While state hospitals across the country continued to close, and their residents were displaced, the new outpatient centers were unable to keep up with the demand. The following photographs show York Hall. (Courtesy of the Leo P. Ostebo Kings Park Heritage Museum.)

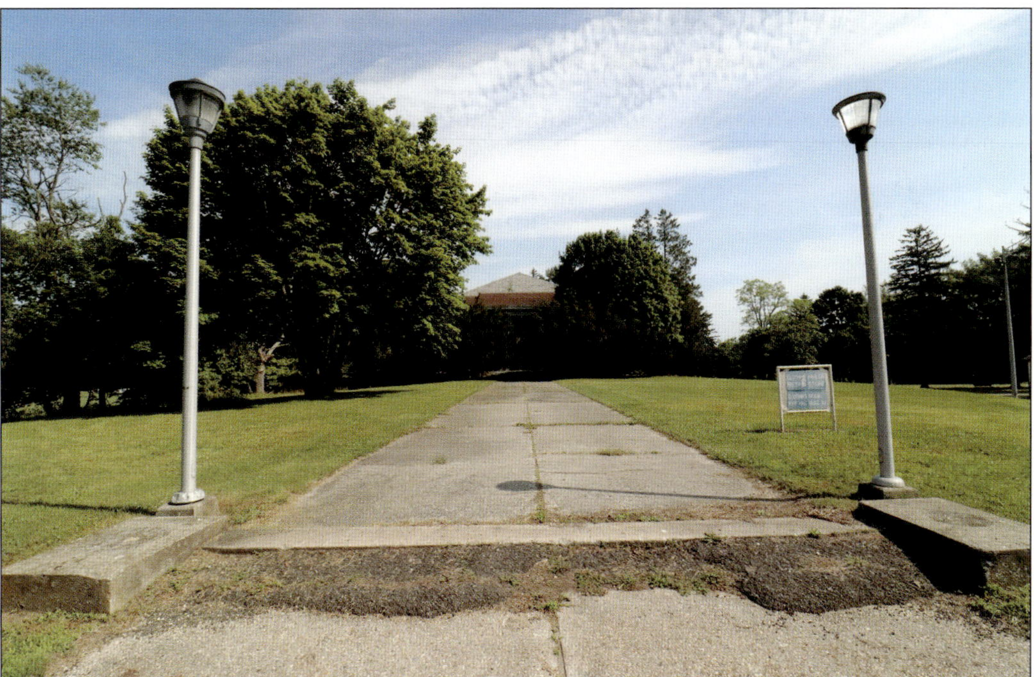

Even the community centers that had opened were terribly underfunded and often unable to offer the type of care patients needed. Nationwide, these souls became forgotten and/or lost in the system. While the public was outraged, progress in finding a suitable solution was slow.

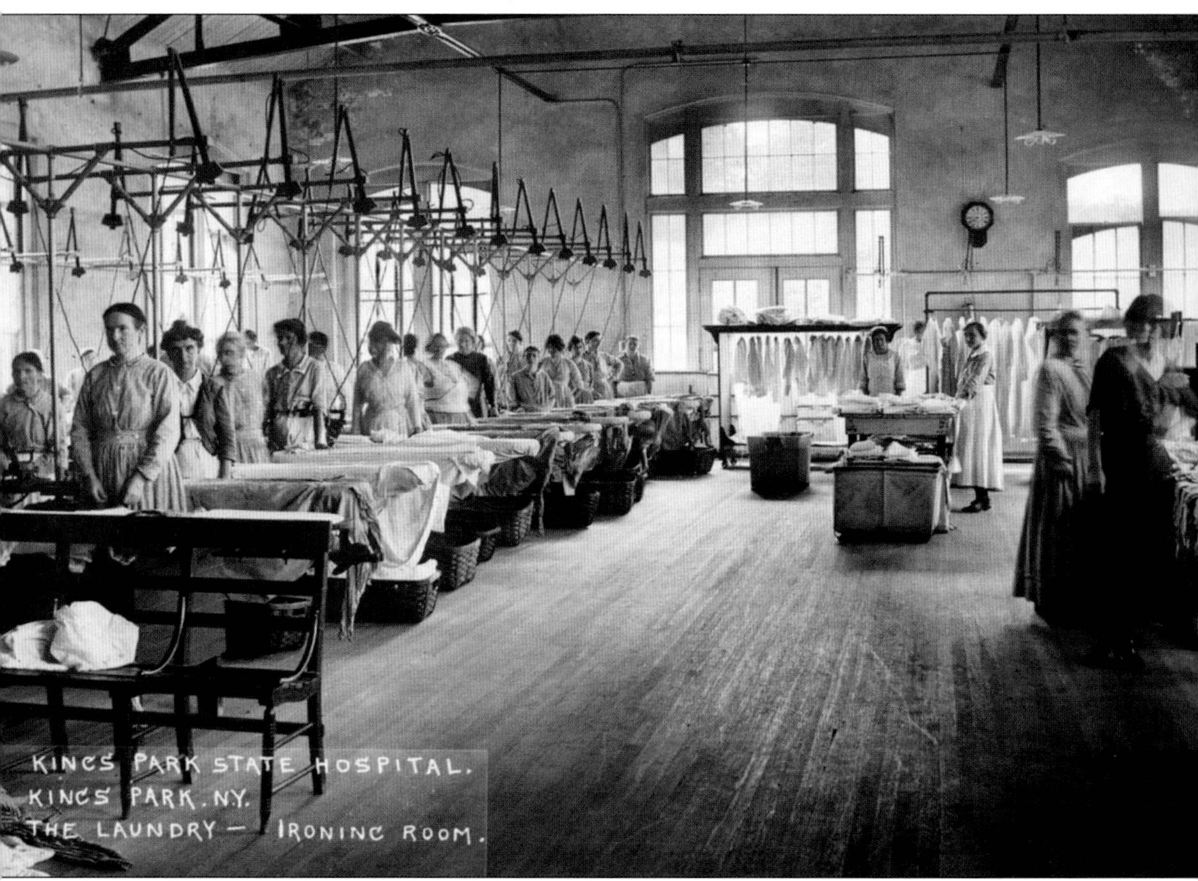

In York Hall, women worked in the laundry and ironing room. Opened in 1885, the Kings Park center transferred its remaining patients to Pilgrim Psychiatric Center or released them, and closed its doors for good in 1996. In 2003, the state put 370 acres of the former Kings Park Psychiatric Center on the auction block. While the asking price for this expansive property was only $2.5 million, there were many drawbacks to the deal. (Courtesy of the Leo P. Ostebo Kings Park Heritage Museum.)

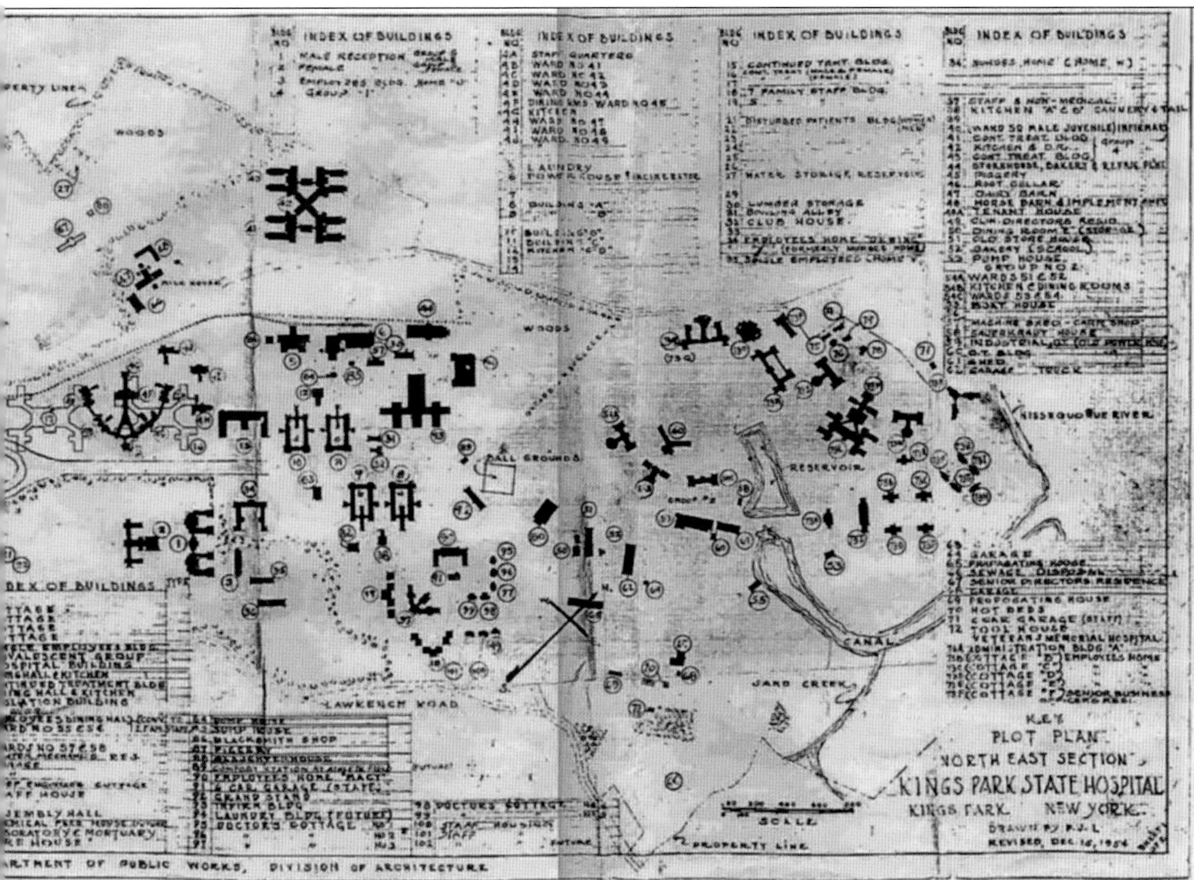

This is a map of Kings Park Psychiatric Center. The first issue for a buyer would be the massive cleanup and the monumental cost of it. Estimates at the time the property was offered put the environmental cleanup cost at about $34 million. While that figure may seem staggering, that is not the biggest challenge. While the property spans 370 acres, most of that is set aside for the preserve, leaving only about 90 acres to be developed. (Courtesy of the Leo P. Ostebo Kings Park Heritage Museum.)